Men, Grief, And Solitude – A Different Perspective

Leo,

I share this book w/ you as a token of the friendship + professional colleaguiality I feel w/ you. Thank you for your care & support.

Your friend.

Dan

Men, Grief, And Solitude – A Different Perspective

Daniel R. Duggan

Solitude Publishers LLC
Alexandria, Virginia
solitudepublishers@gmail.com

Men, Grief, And Solitude – A Different Perspective

Front cover photo by Kristin Duggan.
Back cover photo by Jan Duggan.
Design of book cover by Monica Ripplinger Bagley

Solitude Publishers LLC
    Alexandria, Virginia
    solitudepublishers@gmail.com

Duggan, Daniel R.
    Men, Grief, And Solitude – A Different Perspective
    ISBN 978-0-9908258-0-7
    1.   Grief.   2 Gender.

Library of Congress Cataloging-in-Publication Data
Duggan, Daniel R., 1949-
    Men, Grief, And Solitude – A Different Perspective /
    Daniel R. Duggan
    First edition, 2014
    ISBN 978-0-9908258-0-7
    LCCN 2014922464
    Solitude Publishers LLC
    Alexandria, VA

ACKNOWLEDGMENTS

I want to acknowledge several people who have joined with me in this journey about men and grief. Fr. Art King, OMI, read and consulted with me in my first version of the book. While I did not want to hear him at first, he persevered and got me off to the right start. Rev. Jim Klosterboer spent time with me on a later version that led to this final version in the family retreat in Iowa. I was a better listener, and he guided me to hear the reader better. Finally, Eileen Jinks helped edit this final version. She brought her editorial skills and sharpened its focus. I am deeply grateful for each of these folks and many others for their generosity and ability to think and write more clearly than I, thus helping me to do the same.

I want to acknowledge my gratitude to my three children, Josh, Whit, and Drew, who each read the book and told me what they thought. Each could resonate with the notions of the gender differences in their experiences. Whit helped to refine the referencing throughout the manuscript. I am grateful to my wife, Jan, for her unconditional support and loving patience in my writing. I am grateful to Marvin and Joy Johnson, and Janet Sieff of the Centering Corporation for choosing to support the publishing of this book, which looks at the role of solitude for men in grief. I want to thank Joshua and Monica Bagley for their help in the final version of this book. They helped me traverse the anxious journey through electronic communication that I encountered.

I want to thank my students who have allowed me to teach about gender differences, and how we use solitude in our healing process. Finally, I want to thank those who have journeyed through their own grief and who have been my teachers as we gave to each other. I cherish those memories and lessons gathered along the way.

What follows are stories of men who show us what masculine grief can look like. I endeavored to respect the confidentiality of those telling their stories, and unless I had their permission to share their stories, I changed some details to protect their privacy.

Daniel R. Duggan
Alexandria, Virginia
November 10, 2014

FOREWORD

This is an important book that will impact your understanding of healing. Let me explain. Our culture tends to see healing often in very narrow and elementary terms. It basically boils down to the belief that if we don't cry and/or talk about a loss, we are not really healing. This book will help you see the extreme limits that definition places on us all.

The reality is that we all heal in very different ways and many of those ways have been misunderstood, ignored, or worse yet, shamed and judged harshly. This is very true for the natural paths that men take. Men's emotional pain may be basically invisible to others. Most people simply can't see it. I know this after spending over 30 years working to understand how men heal and writing two books on the topic. I struggled in those early years simply trying to see and understand how men were healing. My struggle was complicated by the fact that men's emotional pain is taboo. Most people are not comfortable hearing a man's emotional pain. For this reason men find ways to process their emotional pain quietly and in a manner that no one will notice. In other words, it goes stealth. It goes under the radar.

That stealth is deepened due to men being harnessed by the provide and protect role. As Duggan describes this in Chapter 4, Gender Differences and Coping. Men are expected to provide and protect. And a good provider and protector is always seen as independent. Any variance from independence is seen as a shortcoming or failure by both men and women. The obvious result is men avoiding the appearance of dependency since this is connected to failure.

So how do men deal with this bind or prohibition? In many fascinating ways. One way is their tendency to use creative, practical or thinking action as a means to process their emotions. Another very important way – and so often unseen and misunderstood – is for men to go into solitude. But does solitude really heal? The author of *Men, Grief, And Solitude – A Different Perspective* thinks so.

Think back to every major religion and some of its most important figures. Every one of them used solitude as a means to heal. Many would go into the desert for long periods. As with many men, finding solitude was a way to deal with feelings, talk things out, decide what needed to be done next, and engage in relationship, again.

I hope you can see now why I think this book will be very helpful to you in understanding healing. It will take you on a journey in understanding solitude and seeing just how it works and how it heals. It will also give you ideas about how to help others who are healing quietly.

Trust me when I tell you that those people you love who heal quietly will thank you for reading this book. When we understand and accept those around us, good things happen.

Tom Golden, LCSW
Author of *The Way Men Heal* and *Swallowed By a Snake – The Gift of the Masculine Side of Healing*

PREFACE

Men and women grieve differently. In nearly 43 years of working with those who grieve as a pastor and chaplain, I have observed these differences in congregational settings, in hospitals, in family meetings to prepare for funerals and memorial services, and in marital counseling sessions. The traditional grief theory I had been taught – that healing results from people identifying their feelings and sharing them – did not fit everyone. I came to recognize that there are many different doors into the grief process and that often the way men go through the grief process looks very different from the way women do. We will look at some of those doors.

When couples or families fail to understand the differences in grieving styles, it can impact their relationship at a critical time. Through this book, I hope to help both men and women learn new skills in relating to one another during difficult times of loss. I hope to help men hear that their style of coping and grieving is important and natural.

In the mid-1970s, a significant body of literature began to appear dealing with death, dying, and grief. One author proposed the theory that men tend to deny their feelings and all they have to do to heal is talk about their feelings. I found this simplistic analysis and solution incorrect and an affront to men. It prompted me to delve into the issue of how and why men deal with their feelings as they do. It was especially important to discover if, in fact, men have a unique way of dealing with grief. Was there a process that helped men deal with loss and grief that was different from the grief theory presented up to that point?

This book reflects my years of listening to and reporting, both in professional settings and through my personal life experiences, what I have discovered about how males cope with grief. Because many men don't often have feeling words to express their feelings, especially grief, their feelings are often conveyed through the stories they tell. You will hear some of those stories.

The stories at the beginning of most chapters are meant to reflect in some way the themes in the chapter. Sometimes they may simply tell a story and be finished. The telling of it completes it. Most of us, when hearing a story, will want to know more. What we're learning, though hard to do, is how to honor both the story and the storyteller. The storyteller, when finished with the story, may not need to tell more.

The first three chapters offer some background on the anatomy of grief; the anthropological imprint and grief; and socialization, rituals, and the importance of honoring male grief. Chapter 4 looks at gender differences and coping, and chapter 5 examines eight different doors into the grief process. Chapter 6 explores the role of solitude in grief. Chapter 7 focuses on the role of the witness and introduces Stan, a World War II veteran, and his story. Chapter 8 sets out 11 ways to be helpful to men in grief. The final chapter directly addresses men in grief, outlining what you need to know when you are the man in grief.

By shining a light on different ways of grieving, I hope that men and women will understand that there is not one "right way" and will be able to respect differences in how we grieve. If you help men in grief, I hope you can be part of the healing. And, if you are a man, my hope is that you find healing in your story of grief. Welcome to the journey.

Daniel R. Duggan
Alexandria, Virginia
November 10, 2014

TABLE OF CONTENTS

CHAPTER 1   THE ANATOMY OF GRIEF AND THE MOVEMENT TOWARD WHOLENESS

"Into the Valley of the Shadow"

A man came into the ER after an accident at home and died about 20 hours later when he was removed from life supports. He had a wife and one teenage son who were the only ones present when I, as chaplain, arrived to be with them. His parents and several siblings and their spouses arrived later and stood by throughout the ordeal.

When I encountered the spouse and son in the ER, they were frightened and overwhelmed. They awaited news of the man's condition. Initially, I asked what had happened and offered them a chance to talk. The wife talked readily about the situation at home when they found her husband. The son filled in parts of the story before asking to go outside for a while. After about a half an hour, I went out to see how he was doing. At this time, he talked a little more about what had happened. I said that it must be one of the worst nights he'd ever had, to which he simply nodded. We stood quietly for a few more moments. Then I told him I would be inside.

Soon the rest of the family arrived. The father was stunned by the condition of his son, which seemed hopeless. He talked little in those first hours. The family members were supportive, often sitting with or standing by the elder father and placing a hand on his arm or shoulder. At times, he would do the same with them. Two brothers initially appeared quite uneasy being in this setting. At one point, I said to them that I was sorry they had to be there but that I was glad they were for the sake of their family. They nodded, and we didn't say anything more about it. They gradually appeared to be more at ease. They did not talk much, but there was a quiet resolve in their demeanor. They took their turn in the ICU after their brother was transferred.

When the life supports were turned off, each family member took a turn to say goodbye. Most of the men seemed to be strained in their emotions, though they voiced their goodbyes and shed tears. It was clear that they were there for their own needs and to be helpful to one another. It was also clear they were honoring their loved one. The women were more open to their tears, to physical touch, and to support. They, too, were there for themselves and one another and to honor their loved one.

The man's teenage son asked to spend time alone with his father, which was honored. Shortly thereafter, the family requested prayer. I found it interesting that no one individual surfaced to be a caretaker for the family. The women accepted the men's inward, quiet way of coping. Differences in grieving were not an issue but were respected and appreciated. In this family's wisdom, they allowed for what each member needed to help them through this valley of the shadow of death.

Through the whole time, it was striking how comforting the men's calm quiet was to the women, who did not appear to be threatened by the lack of verbal expression of emotions. As for the males, by being accepted, they could with time find the right way to verbalize their goodbyes. They needed to feel safe, and solitude gave them a safe place to sort through feelings and thoughts about their loss.

+ + +

When we have a loss, we grieve. A part of our world has been severed from us, and we experience a feeling of brokenness or tearing within ourselves. The healing process becomes a movement toward putting the pieces of our life back together as best we can to create a new sense of wholeness.

Current grief theory defines the healing process as one of identifying feelings and sharing those feelings with a trusted listener. The helping role is one of offering ways to open avenues for the individual to name and share their feelings. This grief theory fits many people. It does not fit everyone.

However, there are common elements in the grief process, such as suffering, the need for relationships, and finding peace through our spiritual journey. I see the spiritual journey as the movement to and beyond ourselves and finding the freedom to be in that movement. While these may be common ground for us all, they may look very different to each of us as individuals.

Although we typically associate grief with the death of loved ones, we may experience suffering with any significant loss in our lives. In *Necessary Losses*, Judith Viorst (1986) speaks to the different kinds of losses we may encounter including passages, relationships, deaths, possessions, body parts or images, jobs and vocations, roles, wealth, and dreams. We can suffer when we lose someone or something that has been dear to us or has shaped our sense of self, purpose, and hope.

The Continuum of Grief Resolution

The stages in the grief process can be considered as points along a continuum. If we have a forewarning of an impending loss, we may experience *anticipatory grief.* In anticipation of the loss, we begin to imagine what it is going to be like when we are without that person, object, or dream, which can be difficult and painful. We may not be ready to experience the impending loss and grief. Yet we try to anticipate in order to prepare ourselves for the worst. Hospice helps many people with anticipatory grief by giving them permission to speak and act in ways they need to when a loved one is dying.

The next point along the continuum of grief is what I refer to as *immediate grief.* This is the moment when we realize that death or loss has occurred. Whether we were able to anticipate it or not, there is no way to adequately prepare ourselves for loss. What I often see as a chaplain is a sudden overwhelming swell of emotion, shock, or panic at this point. Emotions at this time are raw and unfiltered. If people are given safe environments to do what they need to do with their grief at this point, they will normally be able to continue their grief process in a healthy way as they work to put pieces of their lives together again.

Grief is not over in a few hours, days, or weeks. Normally, dealing with grief takes months or even years to work through. This is *long-term grief* in the continuum of grief. One woman reported that after she lost her husband it was a year before she could invest herself in life again. Even then, she related how she would hear her husband speaking to her with reassuring words. Her case shows how healing takes time. That is the way we were made. It is normal.

Some kinds of losses can make it harder for people to grieve. Parents report that the loss of a child brings a sorrow that never ends. The loss of a child can cause parents to feel disenfranchised from their normal social network of support. Other examples of this type of loss include divorce and death caused by suicide or HIV/AIDS. Disenfranchised grief can complicate the healing process by accenting gender differences in how we grieve.

Often it may appear that men pass through the shock and orientation portion of healing work quickly while the women in their lives continue to be mired in the sorrow of their loss. This is a point of conflict for many couples. It is also a point of misunderstanding between partners when they cannot comprehend the differences in their ways of coping. Either can feel misunderstood, distant, or disenfranchised.

Long-term unresolved grief can be found in the continuum of grief. This is also called complicated grief because other factors in life can complicate and inhibit the healing process. A couple may be experiencing a divorce when the death of a loved one occurs. An individual may have experienced several significant losses during a given year when another loss occurs. A person may carry emotional scars from childhood and be unable to enter into his or her grief. People experiencing post-traumatic stress syndrome have emotional fields that are shut down, which then cause them to shut down emotionally when new threats or losses come close or occur.

Drug abuse inhibits a person's ability to draw from resources within and beyond themselves. If a teenage son loses his mother when he is "pulling away from her apron strings" to become his own man, it may take decades for him to grieve fully.

These scenarios show how contributing factors may cause complications in other areas of the individual's life that may never be resolved until the old grief surfaces and healing begins. Sometimes, counseling and therapy may help the person become untethered from the complications of long-term unresolved grief.

Two Kinds of Grief: The Grief of Regrets and the Grief of Sorrow

We can classify grief into two general types: the grief of *regrets* and the grief of *sorrow*. The grief of regrets does not allow us to heal. It occurs when a person does not do or say what needs to be said or done with a loss, so it stays within the psyche as a wound. This is in contrast to the grief of sorrow, which is healing. The grief of sorrow occurs when a person does say or do what he or she needs to say or do with a loss.

An example of a grief of sorrow is the Old Testament story of King David, Bathsheba, and their firstborn. The baby was dying. King David tore his clothes, put on sackcloth and ashes, and begged God throughout the night for mercy for his child. The baby did not survive. Yet, the next morning when he heard that the baby had died, King David's response was to move on with his daily activities and business. His servants were taken aback by his response and asked him how he could do this. His reply was that he had done what he could do and now needed to move on. His response to the death of his child may seem extreme to many of us, but the story points to the importance of doing what you need to do in dealing with loss.

I learned about this from my father-in-law, Lyle, when he was dying. Lyle was known as a mild-mannered, quiet, committed, and ethical man. He was well thought of. As a son-in-law, I had grown to love him. He was 83 when he died. When he turned 80, he noted that his siblings had died when they were 80. Up to that point in his life, he had been very healthy and active. But then he began to suffer from a painful disease.

When he was hospitalized, his physicians were perplexed about what to do. They offered him surgery; he eventually declined, knowing it had little chance of helping him. He knew that within a few days he would die.

Once Lyle made the decision to decline surgery, his spirits lifted. He gathered his family around him and told them he was going to be all right. He was not afraid to die. He thanked them for being his family and told them that he loved them. He was looking forward to seeing people he had not seen for a long time. There were no regrets for him. This gave his family members permission to thank him for being their husband, father, father-in-law, and grandfather. Words of gratitude and memories were shared, and tears of sorrow were shed.

In the days to come, the family stayed by his side to support him in his dying and to support one another. After the funeral and after the well-wishers were gone, there was still a sense of emptiness and sorrow. But it seemed like we were able to give each other and ourselves permission to share and grieve in our own unique way. Lyle taught us that we could name grief and say and do what we needed. I suspect that he learned that in his solitude.

I learned how to tell family members when I was feeling sad. I could also go out alone to the cemetery and be with my thoughts and say what I wanted to say to Lyle. I learned that I did not have regrets when I named and gave voice to my sorrow. I was saying what I needed to say and doing what I needed to do with my sorrow. I was feeling myself heal, as Lyle had taught me.

While the experience of loss was not new for me, the experience of expressing grief with others was new. In my formation, I had learned not to give expression to sorrow and to minimize sorrow and its meaning. As a result, who or what was lost could not be fully honored. Consequently, I had regrets for not saying and doing what I needed to. This pattern of unfinished business affected other parts of my life: my marriage, family, friendships, and work relationships. It kept me from saying and doing what I needed to in those areas, too.

As I learned how to deal with loss and grief differently in the here and now, it helped me see and understand the deep well of regrets I had within me. It helped me see that I could name these losses and choose to deal with the sorrow attached to each one. Healing could begin.

Those who work in hospice settings often see this type of scenario with dying persons and their families. I remember a time when I, as a hospice chaplain, was called to be with a family who lost their mother and to offer prayer. Three daughters were present, all expressing their feelings. The only son was supportive of his sisters but not verbal when feelings were shared. In time, he became verbal as the conversation turned to recalling memories of their mother and childhood. When they were ready for prayer, they all were able to share their tears as they began their letting go and goodbyes. The grief of sorrow occurs when people give themselves permission to handle grief as they need to.

Grief and Self-Esteem

One of the principles of existential therapy is that self-esteem grows when people see themselves doing what only they can do for themselves. They see themselves as being competent and able to deal with life. Self-esteem cannot be given to us. We must earn it and see ourselves with our own eyes and hearts doing what we need to do. Then we can begin to believe in ourselves.

But grief can leave us feeling low on self-esteem and competence. This was pointed out in a research project conducted by Julie Goebel involving parents who experienced the death of a child (1994). She found that there was little difference between mothers and fathers in their grief scores on the Grief Experience Inventory. In other words, both experienced a high level of feelings associated with the loss of their child. Guilt seemed to be equally high for both men and women. The major gender difference Goebel found was in regard to the Despair scale and Loss of Control scale: Both had the same level of feelings. But one externalized or socialized feelings. The other internalized feelings.

The results of this study reflect female and male differences. Women have an *outward focus* in their coping, i.e., they cope by connecting with others. Men have an *inward focus* in their coping, i.e., they cope by connecting inwardly with themselves and their solitude before moving beyond themselves and into relationships with others again. Men will use solitude to help them relate. Relationship is important for both genders, but where each begins with relationships is different.

Both men and women will experience despair or loss of control to some degree as they grieve. Despair and loss of control put us in touch with our limits. We never get to do or say all that we want to do or say. Acceptance of that aspect of our humanness is a part of grief.

I officiated at a funeral with a very complicated family in which the husband/father had died. The mother was in a nursing home and suffering from dementia. There were several children who were at different places with sorrow, anger, repression, hurt, and regrets. Though the siblings were close, they had not been close to their father. All of this not only complicated their individual grief work, but also complicated their care and respect for one another.

I talked with the family before the service to help prepare all of us. I recognized tensions between them and with the situation. I encouraged them before the funeral service to say and do what they needed to with one another and their father. They did talk with each other and found their own ways to give voice to complicated feelings. They decided to have a time in the service where they and others could speak about their father, which I had suggested.

Not all stories told were flattering. The father had been a tough character at times. Other stories were told about his positive attributes, such as his being the only one of his siblings who stayed with his family, his pride for having fought in the war, his uncanny ability to fix machines, and his knowledge and love of horses.

What was interesting was how these siblings found ways to tell their stories and enter into their grief, which allowed them healing of old and new losses. Some of the males in the family led with telling stories they knew about their father. This was a way for them to build their self-esteem and feel competent. The females tended to share about their relationship with their father, validating their way toward self-esteem. These siblings were not going to be able to deal with everything, but they could begin to take care of themselves as best they could at that moment. It marked a new beginning point.

The Spiritual Journey: The Movement to and Beyond Ourselves

Loss and grief affect the spiritual journey for many men and women. I like to see the spiritual journey as that movement to and beyond ourselves as we seek to express and name what we are dealing with, to cope, and to find meaning in our lives. It is the work of finding the freedom to move to ourselves and confront what is within ourselves. This is work the self has to do.

We are also called to move beyond ourselves and into meaningful relationships with others, life, and the Holy as we understand it. This is the work of transcendence of self and recognizing something greater than ourselves. Viorst (1986) noted that change or movement in life may cause loss and grief, itself. I like to think that the ointment or lubricant that allows movement within the spiritual journey is love. I also like to think that we can go through anything when we know we are loved. When we are not sure whether we are loved, the journey becomes harder.

Grief has an impact upon the spiritual journey of men and women. For some men, it may cause them to come to terms with the relational and emotional side of their lives, so they can become freer to relate to others. For some women, they may have to come to terms with what it means to feel safe with their solitude as they come to know themselves apart from the one they lost. Many widows speak of how they had to learn to become comfortable being with themselves.

+ + +

In our solitude, we learn to move to and within ourselves and to respect ourselves, our strengths and weaknesses, our joy and pain. Solitude teaches us to respect the need to know and relate to ourselves. We learn to value relationship by doing so. Solitude teaches us that we must choose to relate to others – to move beyond ourselves.

CHAPTER 2   GRIEF AND THE ANTHROPOLOGICAL IMPRINT

A long time ago, I noticed that I approached men dealing with loss differently than women. However, I did not understand why. In the past 20 years, I have learned to trust the importance of differences in the way that men and women cope with grief. These differences reflect the respective anthropological gender imprints.

Since prehistoric times, changing circumstances of life and nature have demanded choices from humans. Their choices were influenced by the particular circumstances in which they found themselves, as well as by their own physical, social, and psychological structures. Patterns of behavior were formed. These became the templates from which gender roles eventually evolved. These templates are called the biological and anthropological imprint. We can see these anthropological imprints as part of the basis from which we cope with life and losses.

An Anthropological Progression of Gender Development

The anthropological imprint runs deep within us – deeper than we can fully understand. When we are talking about grief and the anthropological gender imprint, we are talking about a natural and fundamental difference in the way men and women grieve. It is rooted in the initial primal development of the characteristics of gender roles for survival.

Often writers refer to the early cave man and woman as their reference point for how our species began to shape the characteristics of the genders. Anthropologists saw that our species divided tasks for the genders according to the needs for survival, which included building a hearth for the family to be sustained long enough for its children to mature and repeat the cycle. In time, bands of families and tribes grew more sophisticated. Anthropologists have hypothesized that group values arose as groups began to express their needs. At the heart of all of this was the maintenance of gender roles that echoed the cry for survival in the human species from generation to generation.

I believe it's also fair to note how we may see ourselves as a blend of the two genders, as Carl Jung (Campbell 1976) contended. He argued that individuals possess traits of both genders in order to respond to the situations they face. We human creatures have learned to utilize more than one way of seeing, thinking, and doing in order to survive, avoid pain, or attain the desirable. This blend reflects our need for wholeness. When we are whole, we can claim resources from both genders that we need to survive. However, each of us will likely have a proclivity for one side of our gender or the other.

According to anthropologists, there are three basic requirements for survival:

- Procurement of shelter and food
- Protection/defense/attack
- Reproduction

For pragmatic reasons, the human species divided these requirements. Since females by nature are assigned the third role, males took on the first two, with some exceptions. This impacted the biological evolution of the species.

John Moore in *But What About Men* describes an anthropological progression of gender development beginning with the obtaining of shelter, food, fire, weapons for defense, and reproduction (1989). It is likely that early in human development, the duty of procuring shelter was shared between the genders. As need and know-how increased, however, there was a greater need for strength to procure shelter. Thus, the male took on those tasks that required more physical power such as procuring shelter, hunting, and protection, while the female focused on tending the hearth, childrearing, and attending to the members of the family.

Villages, towns, and cities developed. Modern success in this arena has set the genders on a more equal footing because these new building skills required greater intellectual ability. Technology and, eventually, the industrial revolution were born out of this progress. Now the information era poses a new challenge between the genders as women have gained a more equal footing. Men in all walks of life are often left to figure out their role and place as the two genders find themselves competing in the workplace and redesigning roles in the home.

Complicating these new relationships are conflicting rules of competition between the genders. A woman can strike a competitive blow to a man, but it is taboo for a man to strike a competitive blow to a woman and cause harm to one he is supposed to protect. It is a double bind. In the world of political campaigns, men running against men readily level character accusations, at will, against one another. However, we do not see the same degree of readiness for a man to throw such character accusations or slander at a woman candidate. If she initiates the attack, the male candidate still thinks twice about doing the same to her. This is a code of conduct that is hard to shake. We just have to think about recent presidential elections when men and women were running against each other and how difficult it was to argue points of view without it becoming more personal or a gender bias. I must admit that today's political world is perplexing for me in this regard.

A Biological Split in the Genders

Left and Right Brain Split

Gender differences have a basis in our physiological nature. We can begin with the brain. Neurophysiologists have pinpointed where certain mental functions take place. These functions helped early humans cope with threats and to fathom and manage new data. Moore (1989) says of the brain's functions:

> The basic functions of the brain are the processing of information and instruction to act. As the continuous flow of sensory signals is transmitted via the nervous system to the brain, it is monitored and interpreted. If action is required as a result, the brain instructs accordingly. The majority of this activity is connected in both obvious and subtle ways with physical survival. Much of it takes place automatically and so rapidly that we are rarely conscious of its happening. (80-1)

The brain is divided into two parts or hemispheres, each with different functions. The left side of the brain is noted for analyzing, focusing, and linear thinking. The right side of the brain is noted for creative, intuitive, multi-tasking, and relational functions. Many people believe there is a gender preference for the left or right side of the brain. Moore (1989) describes the likely gender differences with regards to functional preferences:

Traditionally, the female's procreative role is unchanging, repetitive, predictable, 'automatic', consistent, programmed, reproductive, etc.... Meanwhile, male procurement and defense/attack roles are competitive, aggressive, questing, acquisitive, challenging, exploitative, unpredictable, continually changing; and they require enterprise, risk-taking, initiative, innovation, invention – all of which the power of visualization is crucial for success. (89-90)

While we as a species also evolved in our intellect, Moore (1989) makes note of the limits of the intellect and its mystery:

There can be no doubt that the modifications did enable the human species to survive, proliferate and gain dominance over all species; but those superior cognitive faculties may now be becoming more of a hindrance than a help. Unless there is a purpose other than survival (to what) success should they be applied? Perhaps there is some 'unnatural' but significant 'higher purpose' in the bifurcated and specialized functioning of the cerebral hemispheres? (89)

Moore is saying that we have figured out how to survive. It seems that he is also wondering with us what else there is for us as a species caught in this bifurcated mind.

The Corpus Callosum
Even though the two hemispheres of the brain hold different functions and processes, they are also closely interrelated. A thin membrane called the corpus callosum lies between the left and right sides of the brain and provides the conductors necessary for communication between both sides. Exchange across the corpus callosum takes place continuously, so that most of the time we feel psychologically integrated and unified in our sense of self. While it is harder to show psychological distinctions between the two hemispheres of the brain, the cognitive dichotomies are more easily distinguished.

Since the corpus callosum is thicker and more extensive in the female, this may explain why women may have a better connection between verbal and emotional skills than their counterparts. According to Golden in *Swallowed by a Snake: The Gift of the Masculine Side of Healing*, men have the ability to make connections between verbal and emotional skills; it often just takes them longer (2000). Thus, males have had to develop other ways to cope with and connect to their emotions.

The two sides of the brain can create tension between the need for security and the pursuit of self-interest. The left side fears consequences and the right strives to fulfill ambition. Moore states that this is where the female has an advantage because her two sides are better integrated. She is, therefore, better able to make up her mind when the two sides of the brain are competing for different needs. "With less circumspection and doubt than the male, she will more readily do either what is expected of her or pursue her desires with determination. She is better prepared to abide by her feelings or give controlled expression to her feelings" (1989, 114).

Males under great emotional stresses often need more time to fathom and process both what is happening and their feelings. Moore says, "Meanwhile, the male, in greater confusion, finds himself having to suppress his feelings or fire off his emotions recklessly.... Given that the competitive and power-seeking right side is likely to be more developed in the male, it is understandable why it is he who, through frustration, has gained notoriety as the willfully aggressive and violent gender" (1989, 114). It is also the difficulty of traversing the corpus callosum that can cause a person to appear narrow or rigid. While the female may accommodate more naturally to the different messages between the hemispheres, the male is more aware of the conflicts between the two and may experience more difficulty in resolution.

In an anthropological or evolutionary sense, the function of the left side of the brain is to secure survival of the group or species. Moore accentuates this by saying, "The overall effect of the left-side learning and conditioning is that the person comes increasingly to rely on it for sense of continuity and certainty" (1989, 84). These are needed assurances in the face of threats and can provide a sense of well-being. Thus, the left side of the brain plays a significant role in coping and bereavement.

The left hemisphere of the brain is similar to a computer that receives external input, memorizes it via the senses, retrieves stored information relevant to a task or response, and stores those responses to be called upon. This hemisphere is dependent upon a linear process in which one part of the process is required before the next can proceed. New input or external information enters, is stored, and can be used or recalled when the need arises. This side of the brain may struggle with new data that does not fit a necessary order. The left-brain function is organic and necessary for basic survival needs and has evolved to help the species in this way. Moore (1989) notes that the left side of the brain is predisposed to actions that can be predicted from data assimilated in earlier processes:

> It can only mechanistically attempt to reproduce what it has done before.... Thus, familiar tactics which have proved effective for self-survival in the past will be repeated on the assumption that satisfactory results previously obtained can be achieved upon by taking the same actions. (83)

The left side of the brain develops more quickly than the right in both genders. The female fetus at five months' gestation is developmentally advanced two weeks ahead of the male fetus and at birth is nearly four weeks ahead. The female fetus has a decided left-brain advantage at birth. However, the male has the advantage in the right brain:

> One report suggests that testosterone present in the blood of both the mother and the fetus is responsible during the fifth month of pregnancy for inhibiting the growth of the left hemisphere.... The implication must be that restraint to the left prevents its becoming too dominant over the more slowly developing masculine-right hemisphere. (Moore 1989, 25)

This is considered possible because testosterone competes with the growth of the left side and stresses it, thus preventing it from growing faster.

The left side advocates for safety and an emphasis on the group versus the individual. The right is slanted toward gaining status and power through vanquishing. It favors an adventurous and offensive strategy rather than a defensive strategy based on fear. The left side, according to Moore, is "cautious through fear of making a fatal mistake; the right will take risk through desire to succeed. The left is conditioned to conform to the expectations and requirements of the group, motivated by fear of disapproval. The right is self-generating and strives to fulfill personal ambition, motivated by desire for individual status" (1989, 83).

The left brain desires to please for the sake of security of the group. The right brain is the seat of competition and ambition. It may override the left brain's caution and use negative emotions, such as anger, to win or achieve success. According to Moore (1989), these biological differences in the brain help us begin to understand female and male gender differences, particularly in the way the genders cope with threats and deal with grief:

The right side has what may be described as a subtler, more wide-ranging and less easily definable role.... It involves exercise of the powers of visualization and imagination.... It involves objective consciousness. Objective consciousness permits detached viewpoint and contemplation, an ability to not be involved in what is happening. This distancing introduces the possibility of modifying habitual, reactive behavior. In other words, it allows some perspective on the established left-side process of linear, repetitive thinking. (85)

It is interesting that the right side of the brain defers to the left when the left is in trouble developmentally. The right, practically, cannot exist without the left and will help to compensate for the left. This cannot be said of the left. It seems to confirm the theory of left-brain dominance over the right and harkens back to the requirement for the survival of the species.

X and Y Chromosomes
Moore (1989), in his review of biological and genetic research, identifies the battle of the X and Y chromosomes. The odds for a female conception are higher than for a male. He notes how at this stage the male chromosome has to compete for its place. He concludes that even at this point of development, the male gender is marked with a competitive nature to not only survive but to exist.

Sam Keen writes about the anthropology of gender development in Fire in the Belly (1992). He claims that as a male he sees himself as a nurturer also, but does not identify it with his anima, which is the natural female orientation in his male character. For him, it belongs to his sense of being a husband, father, son, friend, and male. It does not mean that he is not influenced by the nurturing of a woman. But for him, male nurturing is an expression of him as a male in his own right. He said that when he held his daughter in his arms and they played, he felt like a father who was nurturing and not a mother. I found this to be true in my experience as well.

Prolactin, Testosterone, and Tears

Tom Golden (2000) addresses physical differences between men and women. He states that boys and girls have about the same capacity to cry until around age 12, when their hormone levels begin to rise. From that point on, a boy's capacity to shed tears drops because of a decreased production of the needed chemical prolactin. His testosterone rises and continues to do so until about age 25, when it reaches its peak. Sometime between the ages of 35 and 40, male testosterone begins to lower and, interestingly, the capacity for tears begins to rise.

Many male elders report that between the ages of 40 and 50, they began to notice how readily they could cry over sensitive movies or tender family interactions. By the time they reached their 60s, 70s, and 80s, tears would flow even more easily. I visited a 78-year-old male friend who was recovering from surgery. As we talked about his family, whom he missed, he was tearful. When I asked him what his tears were about, he responded, "I just miss my family. You know, I just seem to be able to cry more as I have gotten older." It can be hypothesized that the increased need for "doing" may be the male's response for the decrease in prolactin and other chemical, emotional, and physical changes.

+ + +

It is clear from what science has shown us that the differences between genders, while primarily anthropological and physiological, also include psychological, social, and familial factors. When any of these factors are overlooked, we may find that we are unable to be helpful or understanding of one another.

CHAPTER 3 SOCIALIZATION, RITUALS, AND HONORING MALE GRIEF

"The Gift of Ritual"

A few years ago I officiated at a service that showed me the importance of "doing" and ritual. A young couple had suffered a miscarriage. They were invited to attend an annual interment service held by the hospital and a local funeral home to bury the remains of fetuses that had been miscarried but not buried by the parents. As the ritual began, the young father seemed to be distant and agitated. It was obvious that he was uncomfortable and perhaps did not even want to be there.

At one point in the service, a small casket with the remains of the fetuses was to be placed in the grave. However, the grave was too small for the casket. The nurse tried for several moments to dig the hole bigger with a nearby shovel, but the ground was too hard. Anxiety was rising in all those present.

The nurse asked the father if he would help. The father picked up the shovel and began to dig. It was quite an effort, even for the father. In time, the small grave was big enough to contain the casket. The young father then went over to the casket and gently laid it into the grave that he had helped dig. This was all done in reverence and silence. Finishing his task, he stepped back to be with his wife.

When the service was over, he turned and looked into his wife's eyes. They embraced and wept in each other's arms. Later, they both expressed their gratitude for being invited.

This young father, finally, had been able to "do" something meaningful to express his grief. His "doing" freed him to enter the core of his grief.

+ + +

Although many of our coping skills have their roots in our biological and anthropological imprint (see chapter 2), the socialization experiences of males and females play a role in how they develop ways to cope with the losses and trials of life. In this chapter, we'll examine how socialization impacts one's sense of gender and the place of rituals. We will also reflect upon grief theory and recognize the place of solitude in grief.

Socialization of the Gender Roles

The families in which we grow up leave a social imprint upon us. Families come out of cultures imprinted by anthropological roots. This is the result of both their unique experience as a family in the present and the legacy of generations before them. We are the product of gender imprints, cultural practices and beliefs, and the unique experiences created in each one of our families. Consequently, individuals receive more than a few messages about how they are to live and cope with the vicissitudes of life, including losses and grief.

Early in my professional training, I chose to enter therapy to deal with parts of my story that were not named or well integrated. I could not remember much of my childhood and adolescence or even events that happened six months before. What I learned in therapy was that if I remembered, I would have to deal with painful memories, including my father's alcoholism and abandonment. While I grew up in a family that did not have the tools to cope with that kind of loss and grief, we did learn how to press on and survive those years. In our numbness, we simply went on and endeavored to live day to day.

My therapist was listening quietly one day as I, for the first time, began to name and "report" some of those painful memories that were part of my family's story. I was learning how both of my parents came from families in which their parents had difficulty meeting their needs in a healthy, differentiated way. In psychological terms, *differentiated* refers to relationships in which people allow each other to be individuals without it diminishing the relationship or bond between them.

After I had been reporting my story to my therapist for a while, I glanced up and saw he had tears in his eyes. His tears alarmed me. I asked him if I'd said something wrong. He assured me I had not. He said that he found what I had shared sad. I was confused because I was surprised that my story could have such an impact on him – a story that I could barely tell myself. Yet, his tears validated me. We did not talk about his or my feelings about this moment, but learning why he cried has stayed with me as a good memory to this day. He was listening to and witnessing my story. This therapy experience allowed me to go deeper into the story of my family's impact on me and to try on other ways of seeing and relating to myself, others, and life.

Families can learn new ways of breaking out of their numbness, too. I became acquainted with a couple, the wife in her 70s and her husband in his early 80s, who had lost their oldest son in Vietnam some 30 years prior. While talking with them, they recalled how the loss caused them and their surviving children to distance themselves from their feelings. This prevented them from hearing how the others were doing and feeling, and kept them from mutual support. They simply did not talk about the loss in those first years.

What helped them to move beyond their isolation as a couple was their decision to visit and offer care to other parents who had recently lost a child. In their area, there were no support groups such as The Compassionate Friends, in which parents who have lost a child gather to support one another. They took the initiative to contact those in need, knowing what they themselves would have wanted but did not receive when their son died. In the company of other grieving parents, they could identify and share their story.

In their small, rural Midwestern town, this couple had several occasions over the years to support others who had experienced a similar loss. It is noteworthy to hear how they described the support they offered. The mother saw herself caring for others through her emotions. The father saw himself caring for others through his quiet presence, which expressed that he also knew what it was like to lose a child. Together, they were a good team. They formed a way of relating with each other in these times that, in and of itself, became a ritual for them.

Men and the Length of Grief Resolution
Bob Blauner (1997) edited a collection of stories written by men who lost their mothers entitled *Our Mothers' Spirits*. A universal theme in his book is the length of time it takes men to finally approach their loss and grieve.

He describes how it takes some men decades to finally come to that resolution, attributing this to the complicated dynamics of the mother/son relationship within the family. Blauner relates these complicated dynamics to the task of individuation from *mother* in order to identify with *father* and form a male identity. Rejection, identity, loss, and failed or incomplete re-engagement could postpone healing for decades.

But he also attributes lengthy grief resolution to a male's independent nature, which could prevent crucial supportive and healing relationships from forming. Nonetheless, these males were a product of their family history and their gender. I wonder also if there was a lack of age-related rituals that could have helped them express grief.

The Reinforcing Role of Rituals

In all cultures, both genders have found rituals to be ways of coping with the trials of life. Tom Golden writes cross-culturally about rituals and rites (2000). Rituals help not only to reinforce values but also to give expression to the painful experiences of life. Rituals become important to males, who often use "doing" to help them find expression, just like the young father helping to bury his unborn baby. Up to that point, he appeared isolated from his wife and the others. The ritual provided him a way to do something meaningful with his feelings of grief.

Rosenblatt, Walsh, and Jackson (1976) in *Grief and Mourning in Cross-Cultural Perspective* and Malidoma Patrice Somé (1993) in *Ritual: Power, Healing and Community* (who describes the mourning practices of his own people, the Dagara of West Africa) note gender differences in grief rituals that are consistent across many cultures. All of the cultures studied use rituals to help men and women deal with loss and grief.

According to Therese Rando (1986) in *Parental Loss of a Child*, rituals are active experiences that give meaning and purpose to someone or something we value. They can be one-time expressions or habitually recurring, such as activities repeated on anniversaries. Rando saw how rituals can give grief a vehicle through which to be experienced (1986, 403-4). She describes six properties of rituals:

1. The opportunity for the bereaved to "hang on" to the deceased without doing so inappropriately or interfering with the grief work
2. Assistance in mourning and in confronting unresolved grief
3. The opportunity for learning gained through doing and experiencing
4. A structure for ambivalent or nebulous affect and cognition
5. Experiences that may allow for the participation of other group members
6. A structure for celebrations of anniversaries and holidays

Rituals can reflect the uniqueness of an individual or family. When my children were small, I had the task of putting them to bed. It was my special time with them. Our bedtime rituals included getting washed and dressed for bed, reading a story, my telling a story about "when Daddy was a little boy," and then saying prayers. In our prayers we gave thanks for everyone in our family and named each person including immediate family members, as well as grandparents, uncles, aunts, and cousins. When family members died, we would continue to name them. Often we would pause and talk about them or tell a story about them. This became a meaningful way to remember, to feel, and to stay connected. This experience taught me the importance of ritual for children, too.

Rituals have served cultures and groups to define gender identity. Rituals go to the core of our identity, to what is important to us, and to what we are missing. Robert Bly in *Iron John* (1990) claims that a man's grief for his absent father is a crucible in his identity and ability to cope in later life. In contemporary society, there may be few rituals for many men to claim male identity passed from generation to generation. Yet, Sam Keen argues that it is only one of the critical factors in male identity (1992). Keen contends that a male loses greater identity in trying to meet or fulfill the expectations of "WOMAN" during passages of life (1992). Rites and rituals mark those passages. Keen writes:

> ...the most important rites are those when we separate from the opposite sex to learn the mysteries of our own gender and when we return to join in the marriage and create new life.... The rites, rituals, and ceremonies that marked the transition from boyhood to manhood differed from tribe to tribe and culture-to-culture. But amid all the variations...the passage to manhood was a drama with 3 acts: separation, initiation, and reincorporation. (1992, 28)

Such rituals and ceremonies enable boys to discover manhood and to take up the mantle of new responsibilities including needs for food, shelter, and safety, as well as trust and fulfillment of self, others, and the next generation.

The Loss of Rituals

There are few such rites or rituals in Western culture today for males in their development. Keen's (1992) writing is in agreement with Doka (1989), who maintains in *Disenfranchised Grief: Recognizing Hidden Sorrow* that rituals of passage have been reduced, if not eliminated, for many males in modern culture. As a parent who sat through many of my children's sports events, I have wondered if the wave of over-involved and over-functioning Little League parents isn't a subconscious reaction to the loss of those rites, rituals, and ceremonies. Perhaps by participating in their children's activities, parents are vicariously trying to restore those rites of passage that they missed. There certainly seems to be a lot at stake for many of those parents.

This lack of socialized rites of passage places many males at risk. They may have few resources within, as well as beyond themselves, to deal with the transitions in life and the trials they face. Keen observes:

> When men who have spent their formative years in extroverted action first turn inward toward the unknown territory of the soul, they soon reach the desert – the vast nothingness. Before rebirth comes the painful awareness that we have long been dead. Before feeling comes the dreadful knowledge that we have been anesthetized and are numb. (1992, 234)

My sense is that Keen was identifying the isolation that a man can feel when he goes within himself and discovers that he has cut himself off from parts of himself and his life.

Sometimes rituals are subtle and may get overlooked. Men often have a way of receiving another man's feelings or affirmation without an overt acknowledgment. Listening in silence is one of the rituals that men utilize. You may see a man touch someone on the shoulder, give a look, or just offer a quiet, un-interrupting presence.

The Meaning of Bereavement and the Core of Grief

Bereavement involves the way we grieve something or someone who is taken away from us. It is the process we undertake to cope with the pain and to find the healing that allows us to deal with the loss. Grief consists of those feelings and dynamics we experience within ourselves following such a loss. We know that any significant loss is shaped by our own unique experience of it, including the accompanying feelings, thoughts, and meanings that it holds. This is the "core of grief." At the core of grief is pain. Mourning is how we socialize or express our grief.

In her first book, *Beyond Grief: A Guide for Recovering from the Death of a Loved One* (1989), Carol Staudacher wrote from the point of view of traditional grief theory in Western culture. After its publication, she heard men ask her to write about grief in a way that they could understand. She was puzzled by their request but heard a yearning in their voices.

In her second book, *Men and Grief* (1991), Staudacher described her journey into men's stories and how she came to write about their grief. She was surprised to find a picture of healing that did not reflect the grief theory she had learned. It was here that she did something very important. Because there was little in the literature on the subject of men's grief, she looked for accounts of men describing their own grief. She reported men's stories and allowed them to speak for themselves so they could give their own message and share their wisdom. She did not edit or editorialize. However, she could claim that everyone had to go through their core of grief, but men and women, as she discovered, seemed to have different styles of working through their grief.

I noticed this difference many years ago but was unsure what it was about. When working with a woman who dealt with a loss quietly, my response was often to inquire how she was feeling. Giving her an opportunity to express her feelings usually seemed to help her cope. But when working with a man who was dealing with a loss, asking about how he was feeling did not work as well.

Men seemed to have another style that worked for them, a style that I needed to trust. When a man was non-verbal or focused on "doing" instead of "being," or seemed distant instead of relational, I gave that individual space. I came to understand that "distancing" might be a man's way of seeking solitude. I began to sense that in those situations, the individual was doing what he needed to do to initiate his grieving process.

I remember once making an effort to be empathetic with a young man whose mother was dying. At first glance, he seemed distant and unemotional. As a way of inviting him to be open with his feelings, I asked him if he was feeling sad. He replied dismissively, "No, I'm doing OK." So I excused myself. In retrospect, my perception of him was mistaken. I wish I would have approached him by offering space for solitude, storytelling, reporting, or doing, depending upon his need.

This shift in my attitude and approach also applied to women who needed solitude to cope with their grief. I did not fully understand, but I sensed there was something important happening in the way they were coping. What they were doing seemed to contradict the theory base that I depended upon. That theory base reflected a bias that such things as being distant, resistant, "doing"-focused, and non-verbal were not helpful in the healing process.

A young woman was going through a painful divorce. She stated that she needed people around her at times when she felt lonely, but also that she needed her "quiet time" for feeling and thinking. She found she could best deal with her pain in her quiet time. Yet, the quiet time could also be the loneliest for her. Paradoxically, when she was alone she could touch and embrace her deepest pain. She reported that during these times she found new strength to pass through this valley of the shadow of sorrow in her life. She proceeded toward healing using a style that felt natural to her. The young woman had the wisdom to trust her own coping skills.

Some people report an even more distinct need for quiet time, in the form of "crawling into their cave" or getting away. One man who had lost his job told about how he had been in quite a "funk" until he decided to take a weeklong hiking trip into the mountains. He knew how to survive there, but he did not know how to survive without a job. The solitude of the mountains and the challenges he faced renewed his connection with himself, his fears, his strengths, his hopes, and the resources within and beyond himself. The journey was a ritual that he had used before when he needed to name and manage chaos and uncertainty in his life.

Honoring Male Grief

I have learned to *honor* gender differences the older I get and the more I study and appreciate the human person and community. As a child of the baby-boomer generation, I can look back and see how I rejected my male side when I was a young man. Now, like many men at this stage of life, I have wondered just what I rejected. I identify with women who tell of longing for a part of themselves they felt was not acceptable and which they gave up in order to be more acceptable.

What I rejected was the traditional image of male that was motivated by acquisition, power, dominance, war, individualism, paternalism, and constriction of emotions. But what I replaced it with reflected more of the other side of myself, the feminine side. This I saw as the nurturing, emotive, and connected side. Throughout my 20s and 30s, this was my new ideal self. But by my mid-40s, I was beginning to feel a strange and disconcerting loneliness. I was beginning to wonder what was missing, what I had rejected.

In retrospect, it is easy to say that I had not been wise enough to discriminate between what I wanted and did not want to keep. I had done some psychic harm to myself. A part of me was beginning to cry out for healing and reconciliation.

Keen (1992) describes a healing experience in his own life following the loss of his father when he was 33. It was his first acknowledgment of grief in his life. He was involved in a therapy group in which he reported his story without interruption and was able to express his grief in his own way:

> Since boys are taught not to cry, men must learn to weep. After a man passes through arid numbness, he comes to a tangled jungle of grief and unnamed sorrow. The path to a manly heart runs through the valley of tears.... I was thirty-three years old when I shed my first manly tears. On the day my father died, the dam burst and I lost control of myself. From the first awful phone call until after the funeral I was awash in grief. It was the first time my wife saw me cry. I soon regained the semblance of control, and when I was in danger of weeping, left the house and went on long walks. Four years later, I was telling a therapy

group about longing for my father to return from his long trips when I was a boy when, without warning, I erupted in an orgasm of grief. Wave upon wave of sobs followed, gathering up all of the pain of my life into a crescendo. I cried for the boy who missed his father's arms, the young professor who already felt old and burdened, and for the man who one day would die and never know why. When I finally stopped crying, I felt empty and embarrassed. What would 'they' think of me? Certainly they would not respect me any longer since I lost my cool.... To my surprise I found many had tears in their eyes and they looked at me with unbelievable but undeniable tenderness and compassion. (134-5)

Keen is writing about his manly tears, but we know that boys, while "taught not to cry," also lose some of the chemical makeup necessary for the production of tears upon puberty, as explained in chapter 2.

Neil Chethik (2000) researched how males of all ages dealt with the loss of their fathers. He observed that most men avoided grief counseling because it did not fit them. "Most of the research thus far has focused on how women handle loss. Thus, it's no surprise that affective expressiveness – especially crying and talking about the loss with others – has come to be seen as the accepted norm for grieving. Those who cope with loss in other ways are often considered to be doing it 'wrong' " (Chethik 2000, 4). There are men who report that they don't go to a therapist to deal with their grief "because the therapist will try to make me cry," as a 34-year-old man said to me when discussing the loss he had. Men often use a way of grieving that involves dealing with cognitive processes, managing emotions, and doing (Doka and Martin 2000; Chethik 2000).

We are clearly learning that men have another method of coping with grief. Research conducted in the mid-1990s revealed that men might possess a different way of grieving that is often just as effective as that used to support the feminine gender (Moss, Moss, and Rubinstein 1996-97). Moss, Moss, and Rubinstein's research included 43 midlife men who had lost elderly fathers. In one of their key findings they stated, "...the male orientation [toward grief] is essentially adaptive. Rather than leading to a vulnerable self, action-oriented coping may enhance immediate mastery and bolster self-esteem. A cognitive orientation to loss may better enable a long-term processing that is slow and incremental rather than sudden and jarring. (1996-97, p. 273)."

For instance, males dealing with the death of their fathers might become outward-focused and attend to funeral planning, support of others, or keeping track of things that needed to be done. Others might focus inwardly as they try to make sense out of their loss such as rationalizing that the death might have been for the best, or "He gave a good fight." The surprise for these researchers, Chethik (2000) noted, was that these ways of dealing with grief seemed to work.

Kenneth Doka in *Disenfranchised Grief: Recognizing Hidden Sorrow* (1989) writes that men are often in a double bind in their grief work. They are wired to use solitude to help them grieve. But when men are ready to move beyond their solitude, they enter a culture that has lost many of the rites and rituals that formerly enabled men to "do" or "work" through their grief. They are expected to be "manly" and not express their feelings or cry openly. They appear to suffer in silence or to become stoic or without feelings.

Sometimes we infer that the person who uses solitude or silence to cope with grief has a *defective* way of grieving. I want to emphasize that solitude is not isolation but rather a place where we go to relate to ourselves, to what has happened, and to what is meaningful to us. Men seem to be wired to go there when faced with a deep loss.

I have often seen this in the hospital setting when there is a death and family members are present. Women may gather and talk. Men may stay on the fringe, find some space alone for a while, or stay with family but remain silent. Staff may interpret that the men are not supportive or that they need help because they don't know how to be with others and/or don't know how to talk about what is happening. In some situations, that may be true, but it is not true in all cases. What is true is that men are often ignored or not honored for the way they grieve or for what they have to offer.

+ + +

What we have discovered here is that socialization, particularly in our family of origin, and the use of rituals have an impact on how we grieve. We have pointed to the importance of honoring the differences between men and women in how they do their grief work; these differences are the focus of the next chapter.

CHAPTER 4   GENDER DIFFERENCES AND COPING

"Two Brothers and a Sister"

A father of three grown children, two sons and a daughter, died in the hospital. The older of the two sons, a local shopkeeper in his late 30s, was the only one present when the father died. The son practiced a faith that wasn't open to other faiths, so had declined an earlier offer by the nurse to call the chaplain. But when the father died, the son requested a chaplain. The nurse and the son were present when a student chaplain and I arrived. The nurse was removing tubes and attempting to make the patient more presentable.

The son stood stiffly a few steps from the foot of the bed. He busied himself with details of the room. He particularly wanted the curtain drawn between his father and the door so people would not be staring in at his father and was relieved when we did so. We remained for about 10 minutes. It was obvious the son wanted to leave the room, so we excused ourselves, saying we would return in about 30 minutes when other family members were due to arrive. The son left the room with us and walked quickly to a small waiting room where he could be alone.

The second son and the daughter were walking down the hallway when we returned. The older son was waiting outside the room. After introductions, we walked into the room together. The second son and daughter approached their father, whereupon the son bent down and kissed his father's forehead and told him he loved him. The daughter stood motionlessly by him. The first son, a few steps away, was in his spot on the other side of the bed. Now he was reporting to his siblings on what had transpired up to this point. They began to share some stories, beginning with, "Remember when..." The daughter, though quieter, also shared memories. This lasted about 10 minutes, at which point they all left the room. The first sibling went to "his room" at the end of the hallway. The other two went outside for a smoke.

We chaplains returned in about 25 minutes. The siblings were sitting in the room, sharing stories, and answering questions for the nurse when she came in. After about 25 minutes, I offered to share a prayer, for which they seemed appreciative.

This story illustrates gender characteristics and reminds us not to make assumptions based on gender. It shows the importance of allowing the other person to teach us how to be with him or her in grief.

Male and Female Identity

In her pioneering book, *In a Different Voice* (1982), Carol Gilligan observes that in Western culture women and men appear to have different core needs based on their gender identity. In addition, these identities give both genders stability, meaning, and self-esteem. Gilligan writes that identity for the feminine gender is centered in the need to be "connected" to people. For the masculine gender, the need is to have a "separate" identity and to have this individuality and autonomy accepted.

In times of health and relative balance, men and women with different sets of needs draw strength from one another. In times of trial, such as a pregnancy-related loss, the presence of men and women in the same room could be more like salt in a wound. Gilligan (1982) stresses how much men and women need each other in their lives. She also notes how women and men wish that the other could be more like themselves in the way they cope. Different styles of coping present at the same time can complicate healing. Even when people are accepting of differences in the midst of loss, differences can be painful. When couples experience a loss, both individuals may have their own avalanche of feelings and yearn for people like themselves to help them cope.

While contemporary grief theory identifies that healing begins when talking to others about grief, that step can be intimidating and counterproductive to men, who often have a different way of entering grief. The expectation that a man should talk about his feelings may serve to drive couples apart, driving the male deeper into his cave or inner self.

Another perspective on the healing process is found in Carol Staudacher's *Men and Grief* (1991). She writes about a style of grief work that is characterized by a man going within, seeking inner solitude to get in touch with himself and what has happened in order to begin to heal. She helped me see this as a kind of sacred ground for the man. The person goes inside to tend to his wounds. When enough healing has occurred, the man is strong enough to leave his cave or place of solitude and to enter relationships with others again or even to invite another person into his cave.

Reporting/Storytelling/Doing

Staudacher (1991) identified characteristics of those who use a masculine style of grief resolution. First, men may express themselves most easily in "reporting" or "storytelling."

While talking about feelings may not be natural, talking about the what, when, and where may be more comfortable. And when a listener takes the time to hear such storytelling and reporting, he or she discovers that the words are often colored with emotion. Existentially, in the here and now, these men talk about what is core to them at the time.

As a listener, I have had to learn that asking, encouraging, or challenging a man to grieve another way isn't helpful. What is helpful is letting him tell his story in his own way. None of us, when we are in distress, is inclined to do what is unfamiliar or uncomfortable.

Grief work may also be expressed by "doing." Men, particularly in our culture, have been socialized to be goal-oriented or task-oriented. Men may see their worthiness in doing and providing for their families, but death can strike a chord of failure in fulfilling this anthropological role. In response, they often try to regain esteem in the little things they attempt to do for their loved ones. Rituals can fulfill the need to do something purposeful. Such doing helps to re-create a sense of hope for those whose worthiness and competence are injured by feelings of failure in the face of death.

Tom Golden writes about how he and his brother made a box from wood and tools found in their father's shop that served as the burial urn for their father's ashes (1995). This activity came to hold meaning for them; it was a way to honor their father and their feelings of grief. In centuries past, it was often up to the men to make the casket, dig the grave, or build the funeral pyre. These rituals helped men "do" their grief work.

In Scotland, when a family is gathered by the graveside and the casket is lowered into the grave, the men reach down and grab a handful of soil and throw it onto the casket as the minister says, "From dust to dust and ashes to ashes we return." This ritual allows them to do something meaningful that expresses the pain of letting go. A similar practice may be observed at Jewish burials, where those gathered may pour a shovelful of dirt into the grave.

Categories of Male Grievers

Neil Chethik (2001) in *FatherLoss* identifies four categories of male grievers:

- Doers
- Dashers
- Delayers
- Displayers

Doers are the most common (about 40 percent) and cope by doing meaningful things. They often repeat over and over their story or activity, which over time serves to quiet the powerful grief they feel inside.

The other three categories each represent about 20 percent of the men studied. The *dashers* move quickly through the event of loss, often using an intellectual or philosophical approach to put it in perspective. A dasher might say, "Dad lived a good long life and would not have wanted to continue this way. He would have been emotionally ready to move on." The *delayers* do not exhibit a strong emotional reaction to the death in the short term. Eventually, months or years later, they find themselves returning to their grief and its pain. Chethik observes that typically the loss of the father was the first major loss for this group. The *displayers* show their emotions of grief including sadness, anger, and fear.

Twenty percent of those interviewed by Chethik said that tears and voicing their feelings were core to their dealing with the loss of their fathers (2001). That percentage may have always been consistent, but it will be interesting to watch the present and the next generation of young men to see if this percentage remains the same. The importance of identifying how we cope is found in the influences that change our response to grief and loss and how we move into and through the core of grief.

Gender Differences in Relationships: Gender-Related versus Gender-Specific

The volume of literature has grown during the past three decades concerning gender differences in our culture. Most writers conclude that differences are gender-related versus gender-specific. *Gender-related* characteristics refer to characteristics that may apply to either gender. *Gender-specific* characteristics apply to a specific gender. As a result, each of us may possess characteristics on both sides of the gender chart. Carl Jung was an early proponent in the Western world of the idea that we possess characteristics of both genders within us. Eastern philosophies have understood this for a long time as expressed in the Chinese concept of yin and yang.

The following gender chart describes the primary characteristics of men and women regarding relationships. It is not gender-specific nor is it meant to describe all men and all women. Rather it is gender-related, meaning that these characteristics tend to align with one gender or the other as in a bell curve. This chart outlines some of the gender differences noted by authors in grief literature and from my own work. Recognition of these characteristics helps in understanding the differences in styles of coping between the two genders.

Gender-Related Differences in Relationships

Feminine Characteristics	Masculine Characteristics
• Rapport or feeling talk	• Report talk
• Sharing feelings and relationships	• Storytelling: who, what, when, where, how, and why
• Wants to be listened to and understood	• Wants to have their story witnessed; doesn't need to be understood
• Egalitarian or flat in their social structure	• Hierarchical
• Handles several goals at once and has a broader perspective	• Keeps to one goal or task and is more narrowly focused
• Relational/being-oriented	• Task/doing-oriented
• Tends toward the nurturer, co-creator role identity	• Tends toward the provider, protector/warrior, progenitor/creator role identity
• "Connected" identity	• "Separate" identity
• Moves into relationship to cope	• Moves inward to cope

Gender-Related Characteristics: Feminine

Rapport or Feeling Talk

Those who reflect the feminine gender style communicate by developing a rapport with those around them. Developing rapport gives one a feeling or sense of connection with the other. In both genders, there is a need for connecting with others like oneself through a common language and communication style. For the feminine gender, rapport is characterized by relating through and connecting with emotions.

Sharing Feelings and Relationships

What we are looking at here is the communication style or vehicle that helps to foster relationship. Whether talking about family, work, or whatever is important, those of the feminine gender style filter their talk through their feelings and the relationships they have. When two women are sharing about their day, they typically share their feelings about what has happened. This reflects the ability of many females to use feelings to communicate with one another.

Wants to Be Listened to and Understood

Those who reflect the feminine gender style want to be listened to and understood – that is, they want to feel that the listener "gets" them. They may talk about their feelings or a particular subject in several different ways until they feel they are understood.

Flat Social Structure

At times, women tend to be more comfortable when their social structure is flat, with little hierarchy. Heim and Golant (1992) write about how women tend to prefer less hierarchy, especially in the work setting. When a woman in the workplace receives a promotion, other women may feel, as she rises above them, that she can no longer appreciate the ways women have of working together.

Multi-tasking

Women seem to be more geared to handle several tasks simultaneously and may consequently appear "scattered" to observers. It is like the stereotypical cartoon showing a woman in the kitchen, stirring a boiling pot, with a baby on her hip, a phone at her ear, and telling the child across the room to climb down from the table. Her husband is depicted standing at the kitchen doorway with a bewildered look on his face and both hands on his head, exclaiming, "Agh!"

Relational/Being-Oriented

This characteristic reflects how a woman may respond to what she is experiencing. When she senses a need in another person, she may respond with empathy or by "being with" that person, engendering a sense of "holding" the other emotionally. This relational or being-oriented manner can be important to healing.

Nurturer/Co-Creator Role Identity

As women tend to be more relational and being-oriented in their identity, this leads to a nurturing and co-creator role or identity. Relating to and nurturing another as needed is a building block in a woman's formation. Gilligan (1982) observes that women tend to feel more fulfilled and secure when they feel connected in the important relationships in their lives. When the connectedness is broken or inexplicably changed, anxiety may result.

Additionally, a woman may find a sense of well-being in co-creating, collaborating, or working through a problem in a mutually satisfying manner. This can serve to reinforce her sense of self-identity and self-esteem, especially in difficult times.

"Connected" Identity

For Gilligan and others, a female's sense of connected identity is deeply rooted in her formation, culture, and anthropological imprint. Gilligan writes in *In a Different Voice*:

> Given that for both sexes the primary caretaker in the first three years of life is typically female, the interpersonal dynamics of gender identity formation are different for boys and girls. Female identity formation takes place in a context of ongoing relationship since 'mothers tend to experience their daughters as more like, and continuous with, themselves.' Correspondingly, girls, in identifying themselves as female, experience themselves as like their mothers, thus fusing the experience of attachment with the process of identity formation. (1982, 7-8)

Moving into Relationship to Cope

Under stress or great loss, the feminine style of coping is marked by a movement toward relationship with others who can support, nurture, defend, and attend to them in their vulnerability. This helps to explain the mainstream counseling and therapy approaches that have been developed and applied in the behavioral sciences in the last 50 years. Again, that approach has served many, but not all, people in both genders.

Gender-Related Characteristics: Masculine

Report Talk

Not surprisingly, those who prefer the masculine style may take a different route in developing relationships. They generally use a conversation style that centers on the exchanging of information. It's my belief that when men are reporting they *are* forming rapport. The nuance I am trying to capture is that both genders need that sense of connecting with others like themselves through a common language and communication style - i.e., rapport - but may have different ways of expressing it.

A friend shared a conversation he had with his wife on their way to the funeral of one of his family members. He wanted to talk about how he was doing and feeling. As he told his wife his story, she would interrupt and ask questions. Finally, he asked if she would simply listen because he just needed to talk and be heard. In fairness to her, she was trying to develop rapport by understanding more of his story. He was trying to develop rapport, connection, or solidarity by simply telling his story and having it heard.

Sometimes what appears to be rapport talk or sharing feelings among women does not establish a relationship. On the other hand, through their reporting, men are often, in fact, establishing a relationship even if they're not talking about their feelings. For example, I worked in a small rural town where I often joined a group of men at the local café for mid-morning coffee. Their conversational style was "reporting." They reported on the weather, the price of soybeans, and how much rain had fallen the night before. They knew how to tease and razz each other. But just as certainly, they were developing rapport with one another. There was a sense of well-being present. That's why I prefer to use the term "feeling talk" for the feminine gender rather than "rapport talk." This allows us to understand that both styles of communication, "feeling talk" and "report talk," can lead to rapport.

Storytelling: Who, What, When, Where, How, and Why
This "report talk" is often structured for men. They report the who, what, when, where, how, and why. As Sergeant Friday used to say, "Just the facts, ma'am." What we are looking at is the communication styles or vehicles in the genders that give one a sense of connection with others. I

often say that when a man is telling the story about a painful time or loss, though he may not have or use feeling talk to describe it, the words he uses to tell the story will have feelings "dripping" off them.

Wants to Be Listened to, Doesn't Have to Be Understood
Those reflecting a masculine style may simply want their story heard or witnessed. They may not need to be understood. Telling their story may be enough. Chethik in *FatherLoss* (2001) notes how the several hundred men he interviewed needed to have someone hear their story out and have it "witnessed." It was my sense that they needed to have their story known and that the telling of the story was their way of expressing the feelings they may have had within them. Chethik simply listened quietly as each recounted their story.

Hierarchy
Hierarchy is important in the masculine style because it provides order and a scheme by which the family, group, or community can acquire the expertise needed to survive and succeed. There is order and security for a man in knowing to whom he can turn for help.

When times are good, a man may aspire to climb the competitive ladder, whether in a family, on a team, in the workplace, or in politics. When times get tough, he may look for those in positions of power in the hierarchy for advice and answers. It is not uncommon in a hospital when a family member is brought into the ER for the wife to cope through developing a supportive, relational network. The husband often copes by going to the top and not wanting to talk to anyone else but the attending physician, who, in his mind, is the most competent person in the situation and who can help the most.

Keeping to One Goal or Task

The man who leans toward the masculine style in dealing with grief is often more single-minded, preferring to keep to one goal or task. He may seem narrow-minded. For men, it is more important to stay focused on finishing a task than it is to ask what others are feeling, let alone share how they are feeling.

Task/Doing-Oriented

This characteristic, like the corresponding one for the feminine gender, reflects how we respond or react to what we are experiencing. The male in this case responds with action or a sense of the task that needs to be done. In a stressful situation, he may marshal his energies, thoughts, and actions toward the goal of completing the task or fixing the problem. In emergency situations, this may be crucial to safety or health. Taken to the extreme, it may seem like riding roughshod over feelings.

Provider, Protector/Warrior, Progenitor/Creator Role Identity

The masculine style tends toward the provider, protector/warrior, and progenitor/creator role identity. This means providing for basic needs; protecting others from harm; taking the initiative to form families; and building communities, economies, political bodies, and so on. I have always been surprised by how quickly the papa bear in me comes out when I believed my wife or children or that for which I had worked hard were in harm's way. This is the protector side of identity. In Western culture, this masculine identity is marked by strong individuals with the inner strength to trust themselves in the face of threats. They learn to trust and honor individuality and the strength within that is typically associated with it. This is a relationship – a relationship with self that is trusted and honored.

"Separate" Identity

The male often finds strength and validation in a "separate" identity, meaning that he finds well-being in his individuality and his being able to manage a challenge or difficulty on his own. But even then, he may not see himself alone due to his knowledge that there are those he carries within himself and his solitude whom he can look to in the worst of times. When the male's sense of individuality or separateness is diminished, he may become anxious.

Gilligan (1982) highlights the gender differences related to an identity based on connectedness versus separateness:

> For girls and women, issues of femininity or feminine identity do not depend on the achievement of separation from the mother or on the progress of individuation. Since masculinity is defined through separation while femininity is defined through attachment, male gender identity is threatened by intimacy while female gender identity is threatened by separation. Thus males tend to have difficulty with relationships, while females tend to have problems with individuation (1982, 8).

I am learning to appreciate that while males may need to separate from external social relationships, at least for a time, they possess an internal world with which they can connect, providing them with a host of relationships to help work through difficulties they may face.

Moving Inward to Cope

When a crisis or great loss comes to those of the masculine gender style, their first step may be to move inwardly to cope. A male may go into his cave and tend to his wounds as a way of sorting out what has happened and then work through possible next steps.

Staudacher (1991) observed this as well. She was struck by how men described their healing process in simpler terms than mainstream theory described it. She noted that men often *retreat* within themselves to manage the pain, disorganization, and anxiety caused by loss. By retreating, they can experience shock and disbelief over what has happened. Then they *work through* their grief. This involves confronting, enduring, and dealing with a wide range of grief responses. It may also involve thinking about, talking about, and crying about the loss (often done alone and in solitude) – doing things that bring both self-esteem and meaning to the man. Finally, there is *resolving*. Resolving may include changes in goals, directions, and commitments. As they retreat, work through, and resolve, men in grief are coming to terms with their changing world. They are finding a way to keep going in a manner that has meaning and purpose. Without this movement into one's self, the male may become lost.

Sacred Ground and Honoring

Staudacher (1991) noted how retreating into solitude was, in essence, entering sacred ground. I believe this is crucial to understanding the way in which men handle grief. In fact, I wept when I first read her words because it was the first time someone acknowledged and honored how I felt. It is my sense that a part of what is happening to a man in grief is that he is not only experiencing the need to retreat, work through, and resolve his grief, but also, in so doing, is honoring the one whom he lost.

This honoring makes the loss a sacred experience. By trusting his solitude, a man is entrusting himself into the care of self and others, where he feels safe. Others may include the memories of others, the person lost, or God (or that which is holy for him). Until he can find a way to honor his loss, a man may feel and believe that his loss and grief was to no avail. Honor can help to restore his sense of self-esteem. He will sacrifice his life, anxiety, fear, and so on, to do that which brings honor to those he loves and to him. When I see someone who seems particularly uncomfortable being present during a crisis, I often share with him that I am glad he is present with his family. I believe the statement is a validating one that gives him meaning and purpose.

The Need to Honor Differences

Differences between the way men and women grieve is a recurring theme for couples and families. The differences can be a source of strength or a source of frustration.

There was a farming couple whose young son died. The boy had a chronic disease that would have eventually resulted in death, but he actually died suddenly from a different illness. As the mother's shock began to diminish, she began long episodes of weeping. This frightened and confused her husband, who eventually got angry and told her to get over it. In his mind, they needed to move on and focus on other things that required attention in their lives. I believe that his pain was as deep as hers, but in his identity as a provider and protector, he felt he needed to stay focused on task and could not prolong his mourning by letting himself feel her pain. Here was a case of two gender cultures clashing.

This is not to argue for anyone to express frustration in harmful ways, emotionally, mentally, or physically. However, I would contend that unless we learn to understand and validate a person's frustrations, we will not learn to be helpful.

Another couple was dealing with their first child leaving home for college. In their daughter's senior year of high school, the mother talked often about her feelings with her husband. It was a tumultuous year between mother and daughter. The father reported that he seldom knew how to respond, so he just listened. The day arrived when they took their daughter to college. After saying their goodbyes, the wife chose to drive back home. He described how as they drove away, he "broke down and sobbed like a baby." What was helpful to him was his wife taking his hand and holding it while they drove away in tears. He wasn't ready to talk about his feelings, but feeling safe in the situation, he could shed his tears. It was interesting that once he reported on his reaction, he could move on to report the feelings he had felt.

In the first case, the husband did not know how to honor the differences between himself and his wife, and he blundered. In the second case, the wife gave her husband his emotional space and did not intrude until she was invited. Fears often make a partner anxious, which, in turn, can cause the person to shut off emotions. Thankfully, that did not happen in the second case. The father needed his tears honored and witnessed.

Chethik's research for his book *FatherLoss* (2001) involved contact with 376 men who had lost their fathers. He held the bias that these men would not want to talk about their loss. Only a handful of men actually declined to be interviewed:

> I was often amazed by the level of honesty and openness of the men, most of whom I'd never met before we sat to talk. Our culture seems to draw back from male emotion, especially grief, so I half expected the men I spoke with to be guarded about any personal turmoil that followed the deaths of their fathers. It did not happen. Rather, sitting with these men in their kitchens, living rooms, and backyards, I found them eager to talk. They *wanted* to recall the good times with their fathers; they *wanted* to revisit the death, even when it drove them back to tears. (6)

As I read Chethik's book, I was surprised, too. It was liberating to hear that, given the right conditions, men wanted and needed to tell their story in their own way. All they needed was a witness, a listener.

+ + +

It is important to look at specific gender differences that affect the way we cope. Acknowledging our differences has the potential to give us greater appreciation and understanding. It can also help to demythologize and correct misconceptions we hold about ourselves and others.

CHAPTER 5   DOORS INTO THE CORE OF GRIEF

"A Tale of Two Men"

Ted admitted himself into a local psychiatric unit after a suicide attempt. He managed to put the gun down just before pulling the trigger. He knew he was hurting deep inside. During the last five years, he had experienced several failures in his work life. Each failure sent him deeper into self-doubt and further into a sense of isolation. Each loss represented another step toward an endless spiral of despair.

However, it was not until he was asked in the hospital about significant losses in his life that he connected some of his hurt to his wife, who had died in a traffic accident five years earlier. Six months after her death he decided it was time to move on from "feeling sorry" for himself, so he buried himself in his work. What Ted did not realize was he had also buried his hurt. With his hurt "out of sight and mind," Ted became isolated from an important part of himself.

Bob's story is different. Bob was 77, a widower, remarried, separated from his second wife, very healthy, and still active in his field of work. However, he was recently diagnosed with early stages of Parkinson's disease and was, at first, shaken by the news. After having studied the disease, he determined, along with his doctor, that with odds in his favor he probably had "one good year left" in his life. It was sad and sobering news. Yet, Bob decided that he would make the best of a bad situation.

He decided to enter a year of disciplined physical, emotional, social, and spiritual growth. He was going to stand with his disease and live what time he had left to the fullest, dealing with possibilities and limitations as they arose. His belief was that this "experiment" would allow him to live with integrity and be open to life, and, if he was lucky, might even extend his life. His desire was to do something that would make a difference in his life.

+ + +

What we learn from Ted and Bob is that *doing* can have different outcomes. Ted was blocked in his healing because he did not know how to give expression to his pain. He became cut off and isolated from an important part of him. He busied himself after his wife's death and in effect buried his pain. On the other hand, Bob found a way to begin to deal with his loss of health by determining to make the best use of the time he had. His doing was connected to his loss, which enabled him to give expression to his loss in a way that was meaningful to him.

As we discussed in chapter 3, the core of grief is the deep pit of pain and sorrow that we must engage in and go through to heal from our loss. Numerous doors surround the edges of the core. These doors become the passageways we use to enter the core of grief.

Most people develop preferences for how they deal with loss. These preferences are shaped by many things including gender, psychological makeup, family history, ethnicity, anthropological imprints, and spiritual and life factors. The figure below identifies eight common doors into the grief process.

The Eight Doors

Doors Into the Core of Grief

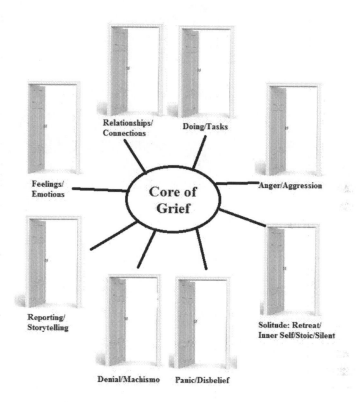

Feelings and Emotions
We know that when men have a loss, feelings or emotions are attached to the loss. Some men begin their grief work by going through the door called feelings. Chethik (2001) characterized men in this group as displayers. Once the initial shock begins to wear off, feelings of sadness, fear, anger, anxiety, and despair may surface enough to be

consciously felt. For some, the natural course is to follow the feelings and find expression for them.

Relationships and Connections

Another door is that of relationships and connections with others as a way to cope. Moving into relationships can provide comfort, support, and a sense of well-being crucial to dealing with the tremendous feelings, dynamics, and disorientation of grief. As we've seen, much of grief theory and therapy is based upon this premise – that when people move into relationships to deal with their feelings, they will begin to heal. That has proven a helpful approach for many people.

Doing and Tasks

Especially for men, doing and finding a meaningful task is another door. Sometimes just being active and doing something is a way to engage and begin to work through one's core of grief. When my father-in-law, Lyle, died, I felt his loss deeply. I picked a large bouquet of wildflowers from his childhood farm home for the funeral. Doing this task helped me to be involved in a meaningful way with the family while giving expression to my sadness.

Some things can only be experienced by doing. You can't learn them by imagining what it is like. Author Ray Anderson called this "sweet agony" (1995, 31). He wanted to learn how to plow with a team of six horses. He was 13. After watching his father drive the team up and down the field, plowing furrow after furrow, he imagined himself with the reins of six horses in his own hands. Finally, one day his father let him take the reins and the team took him down the field.

Ray did all right until he had to slow the horses at the end of the field to prepare to turn them around. It was disastrous.

The horses tangled. The plow got stuck in the ground. His father had already begun the long walk to help. He knew that his son could learn only by doing. After showing him how to correct the problem, he let Ray do it. His father was teaching him how to deal with the turns in life by helping him face them, not by taking them away.

I remember the story of the father who took the body of his three-year-old daughter to a regional hospital across state lines so that they could perform an autopsy on the body and learn about the disease that had taken her life. By crossing state lines, he risked being arrested. However, it was important to him to do this last thing for her and the family.

No one else can grieve your loss for you. You must experience it yourself and in your own way. I do not find it unusual when a couple whose newborn has died wants to take the body from the hospital to the funeral home themselves. In their minds and hearts, no one else could make that journey with their child better than they could. It is something they feel they must do.

Anger and Aggression
Anger and acting out in an aggressive way is another door. Anger can be a way of reacting when one feels helpless. A young man came into the ER and learned that his father had died suddenly. His first reaction was to turn and walk out of the ER, and, on his way out, he banged his fist on the wall. The young husband of a woman having a mastectomy the next day came into her hospital room as she was talking with the chaplain and crying because she was afraid. When the chaplain finished the visit, the husband followed him out, told the chaplain he was upset to see his wife crying, and asked him not to return.

In another case, a father became verbally aggressive with the doctor who came in to report the poor progress of the man's son. The doctor was wise enough to allow room for the father's anger at that time. In another situation, a middle-aged son came to the ER when he heard that his father had had a heart attack. His father died. The son reacted with anger and blamed the medical staff for incompetence. It did not help when the doctor reacted to him with anger, which accelerated the son's anger. Each of these anecdotes depicts men who walked through the door of anger as their first step into their core of grief.

Reporting and Storytelling

Early in a loss, reporting is a way to name what has happened. Eventually, feelings come to bear upon the story as it sinks more deeply into the griever's psyche. One family in crisis whose members are arriving at different times in the ER may see a member of the family taking the lead in reporting to the newcomers. Sometimes, more than one person may share that responsibility. Reporting serves as a way to engage one's grief. This reporting may move the person closer to feelings.

Storytelling can be another function of this door into the core of grief. Storytelling may come later when the shock of the immediate grief has worn off somewhat. People are realizing the magnitude of the death and loss. They are literally internalizing the person they lost and their connection and relationship with that person. At this point, stories and memories often come to the surface. Such storytelling serves to help people remain in their core of grief, which honors who or what was lost as well as one's feelings and thoughts. If this is done in a family context, the family is learning how to be present to one another, as well as learning how to develop a safe and trusting space for each other in their grief.

Denial and Machismo

Freud identified a number of defense mechanisms people use to help cope with anxiety and difficulties. Denial is one. It is used when an individual cannot acknowledge or cope with what has happened. In response, the event is reframed, ignored, or pushed away. A nurse was told that her son had been brought into the ER dead on arrival. Her son had had numerous brushes with death because of his lifestyle, but she did not want to believe that it was her son who was in the ER now. It took her two hours before she was ready to view her son's body and identify it. This was a painful experience for the entire staff, but it was important to stand beside her until she was ready to take the next step for herself. Her denial was helping her to cope with the death of her son and to come to terms with it in an incremental and manageable way.

Denial can be more subtle when used subconsciously to stave off the reality of what has happened. I've witnessed many men at the hospital who come after receiving the news that their loved one has died. They may spend a few minutes in the room with their loved one, sign papers, make a few phone calls, and then leave quickly. Denial for them may simply be holding off the fuller range of feelings of grief, or waiting for a time to enter the depth of their feelings when they feel safer doing so. Men are often taught from boyhood that it is not okay to shed tears. So, when they feel the most vulnerable, they may choose to deny or minimize their feelings. If they can find places where they feel safe and can be with people whom they trust, their feelings will come in their own time and way.

Machismo is another defense men use when standing before their core of grief. The macho stance counterbalances the feelings of vulnerability and powerlessness. Often, feelings can seem out of control. A strong will and fortitude can seem like the best defense for the chaos and disorientation of death and loss. It enables the man to stand at the door of grief and enter as far as he can go, do as much as he can, be a part of the family story, and feel good about his contribution. In a major way, being macho is about self-esteem that has been wounded. Death has dealt a blow to this man's identity as protector of the family, so he stands firm in the face of death.

Panic and Disbelief

Another door into the core of grief is panic and disbelief. One theory of grief resolution shows two tracks that move through several components of grief work including shock, feelings, power, intellect, commitment, and completion. In this theory, a man can move back and forth on the two tracks while moving forward and backward in the healing process. Panic describes his reaction to extreme disorientation, emotionally and cognitively. Because of fear, he flees from touching any reality that would make him name his loss to deal with the deeper pain. Panic involves cognitive dissonance when what has happened, such as a loss, does not fit with what he wanted or planned. Yet panic becomes a step through a door that allows him to enter his core of grief.

The matriarch in a large Italian family was brought to the hospital because she was dying. Family arrived. When the attending doctor came to give the news that she had died, 20 or more of the 30-plus family members looked frightfully at one another and began to scream and wail. Fortunately, they were together in a large room where they could have privacy and support one another. This panic was seen in both men and women.

When this initial phase of grief subsided, they were able to deal with other feelings and needs, including contacting other family members, telling stories, and being ready to have the priest pray with them as they entrusted this matriarch into God's eternal care according to their faith. This family would not have been able to enter as deeply into their sorrow had they not been able to enter through their door of panic.

Disbelief is related to panic because it involves the cognitive part of ourselves. It is similar to but different from denial. While we may use denial to say this event did not happen or is not as awful as we supposed, disbelief is the inability to fit what has happened into our framework of understanding. You may hear the words, "I cannot believe this is happening," or "I cannot believe she is gone." This cognitive dissonance may make it impossible to comprehend the loss as a part of one's life and reality. While the emotions may not yet be accessible, the person is trying to reckon with reality by naming and thinking through the loss to make it fit in a manageable way.

We can often see this in children, who do not have the full ability to understand death. They may give meaning to death in unusual ways, such as a consequence: the child who is afraid to go to sleep because grandma "went to sleep and did not wake up." Adults can struggle with trying to understand what has happened in death, too. It is this struggle that allows them to enter their sorrow through the door of disbelief.

Solitude: Retreat, Inner Self, Stoic, Silent
Through the door of solitude, a man moves within himself to deal with grief. He will often feel more safe here than having to relate to others when too much is happening. By moving to a place within himself, he is often able to slow down what he is dealing with so he can identify it and

discover what has happened. We will explore the door of solitude in depth in chapter 6.

A Door into a Young Man's Grief

The following is the story of a young man who lost his father and found a door into his core of grief. He was 35 years old. He stood alone in the funeral parlor viewing his father. He was numb. He could not think or feel. His legs felt weak, so he placed his hands on the side of the open casket as he looked at his father. As he looked upon his father, thoughts, sounds, memories, and feelings began to flood his inner world.

In those few minutes, a rush of feelings found their way into his consciousness. But as enormous as they seemed, they became fitting expressions that he could carry. In his own time, he would learn when to share what he needed to share with others who were significant to him. But these minutes were precious. As these moments came to a close, the man stood at his father's side and wept. His tears gave expression to his sorrow. He was able to speak words to his father that he wanted to speak. The longer he stayed with his father, the more he knew he was honoring his father with his presence. When he was done, he was ready to say, "Goodbye, Dad."

Several characteristics mark this story in terms of what we could describe as a masculine style of coping with grief. The first is how the young man was alone in solitude with his father with his shock, feelings, and thoughts. This solitude became the door that allowed him to enter his core of grief. The second characteristic is his use of solitude to prepare him to relate again. The third is honoring his father by staying with him long enough to sort through what was necessary. A fourth characteristic is sharing his tears in his solitude. He might not share his tears outside his solitude. For most men, tears are very precious. They choose where and with whom they will share their tears.

+ + +

All of these doors are ways to find expression, name, manage, and give meaning to loss and grief. We may be surprised at other doors that can usher us into our sorrow and grief, such as dreams or music. We can learn to trust them for ourselves.

CHAPTER 6   THE DOOR OF SOLITUDE

"The 'Good Soldier' Son"

A 35-year-old son and his wife had been waiting in the ER for about an hour. His father would arrive by helicopter from a small hospital because it had been determined that he needed life-saving surgery. This was an anxious time as they waited helplessly. Finally, the son went outside, where he remained for about a half hour. The staff was concerned about how he was handling this situation and called the chaplain to help.

I arrived in the ER and greeted the son's wife, who told me what she knew about the father's condition. I asked how she was doing. She seemed comfortable talking about her immediate concerns and worries. She said that her husband was outside. I asked how he was doing. She said she wasn't sure. We went outside so I could meet her husband and see how things were going.

We met him in front of the hospital, and I introduced myself. The son appeared anxious. He said he wanted to see the helicopter come in and wanted to be outside to see his father. He found it hard to talk. After a brief conversation, I let the son know that I would check back in with him before too long. I excused myself and returned to the ER.

Later, I caught up with the son and the rest of the family in the ICU family waiting area. The son took the lead in introducing me to the family. He talked about his father's condition and the fact that his father was already in surgery. Though it was still an anxious time, the son now seemed capable of receiving support as well as giving it. The father survived surgery and lived to go home.

This was a trying time for the couple. They both appeared to handle the crisis in different ways. Initially, the wife remained in the small waiting room in the ER after her husband went outside. She may have wanted to give him space. We can surmise that if he remained, he might have felt pressure to talk when he did not want to. That could have made him feel unsafe.

By going outside to watch, he was actually *doing* something. It was my sense that he was standing guard, like a good soldier for the family, so that he would be ready to let his father know that he was there for him. The wife seemed comforted in being with her husband. Before long she went back inside. Her husband was still waiting for the helicopter to arrive. His words to his father when he saw him were, "Dad, I'm here." The son had honored his father. He seemed to put together his own natural way of dealing with crisis. Later, he was able to receive support from others. But first, he had to go within, trust his solitude, and do what he needed to do for himself. I sensed that he had found a way to be helpful and to stay connected to his family. The son remained an involved member of the family throughout the family crisis.

Solitude and Going Within

Solitude is the work of going into your interior, of relating to yourself, and of finding both what and who are there. It often involves:

- Inner-talking
- Questioning
- Weighing the past with the present
- Wondering what the future holds
- Planning how one will acquire a goal or meet a need

- Having discussions with others
- Sorting out facts to report on
- Acknowledging and feeling emotions
- Allowing successes and defeats to have their place
- Finding the road to hope

Solitude is an experience of being that runs deep within men. From the anthropological imprint, men learn to trust solitude. Many characteristics of his inner self are often shaped by a man's early lessons of solitude.

Solitude is not isolation. For a man, it is often about going into his quiet space, into his "cave" or inner sanctuary for safety to recollect himself. It is about going into an interior place where he can be in relationship with himself alone, where he can recall relationships and good memories that sustain.

In his research on how men grieve the loss of their fathers, Neil Chethik discovered how men tend to hold their memory of loss within themselves (2001). He observed that men find expression in sorting through the experience of loss internally. They tend to do something special to help them express deeply felt feelings. They seek to find meaning to help them put death and life in order.

Solitude begins early in formation. I am reminded of a small child who fell and was crying. His father was watching nearby and decided to wait for about 10 seconds before going to see if he could help. His intention was to help his child learn that his parents would not always be around for him and that he could look within to find strength to face the pain. In Western culture, the movement to preschool and kindergarten propels the child into a new level of self-discovery and autonomy. Some cultures, like Native American and some African tribal cultures, have a rite of passage in which a child is sent into the wilderness to test his ability to survive.

As we look into our journey, we will often find such passages that guided us in one direction or another. Solitude began early in my formation. My father left us three times before I was 10 years old. After the last time, I did not see him again until I was in my early 20s. I was fortunate to have several surrogate fathers. One was my maternal grandfather, who mentored me while I grew up. One summer day after my father left for the last time when I was 9, we were picking apples. I asked Grandpa, "Why did Daddy leave?" He replied that he didn't know, but then told me that I had a Father in heaven who would never leave me and that I could always depend on Him. His reply gave me hope to believe in myself, others, life, and the Holy. It has been a good memory all of my life.

Had I not been able to share my question when needed, I might have experienced an unhealthy kind of isolation. But I also suspect that Grandpa was beginning to teach me about the importance of solitude. He answered my question in such a way that I could take his words back into my solitude. His words became etched in my inner dwelling space, ones I would revisit and find strength in throughout my life. It marked a passage.

Carol Gilligan (1982), in her gender research, wrote that men derive positive self-regard through being separate – meaning independent or autonomous. In fact, not having a clear sense of separate identity can create distress or anxiety. Separateness opens the door to solitude, which nurtures the awareness of connectedness within. The movement into solitude is dynamic, freeing, and healing.

In solitude, we can experience Sabbath or rest. Thomas Keating, a Catholic monk, has said that Sabbath is not a place but a state of being in our inner world (2003). When men are in their solitude, they can let go of external expectations and attend to what is within. Reflecting on solitude, a man once told me, "I'm there to be with me." These are nurturing and healing perspectives.

Some men find that an actual journey into a forest or wilderness helps them to discover their inner world. Andrew Rogness, author of *Crossing Boundary Waters* (1994), contended that a journey into the wilderness enables us to trust ourselves as we are. There we can ask, "Who am I?" and "What is my life about?" A wilderness journey enables us to face mystery, which we do not always do well. Such a solitary journey causes us to listen to our own questions, to ourselves, and to mystery itself. Some Native Americans teach that we should listen seven times to another person's words in our mind before speaking. This is to quiet the soul so it can hear the other's soul as well.

While solitude is not contemplative prayer, Keating says something about contemplation that I believe parallels solitude. He says that contemplation is an inner dialogue between oneself and the Holy (2003). Again, we see the nature of relationship that occurs in solitude. Solitude, then, is a place where dialogue between oneself and what lies beyond oneself occurs. Keating affirms that what takes place in our inner room or sanctuary is ultimately an affirmation of the basic goodness of self (2003).

So we can see why many men explore solitude before turning to relationships when they have been wounded by loss. In solitude, they find the security to face themselves, as well as their despair, pain, fear, anxiety, and vulnerability.

Solitude is work. It is about a journey and a process. When men enter their solitude, it often requires extraordinary effort on their part to stay there. It requires effort to listen and to be honest. Solitude demands openness, vulnerability, questioning, and searching for answers. In solitude, men work to sort out what happened and ask what's next. Finally, men will reach a point where they have to make a choice – whether to invite someone else into their cave, *or* move out of the cave with a new sense of self and purpose, *or* ask for help. In solitude, men make choices about what they believe will lead to their healing.

Solitude as Sacred Space

Sacred space is the inner place where consciousness allows for the array of human experience to be named, validated, honored, celebrated, comforted, strengthened, confronted, and reconciled. Carol Staudacher (1991) reported that she observed and heard in men's own words that they were entering sacred space when they moved into their solitude when they were hurting or grieving.

In a 2006 presentation titled, "Solitude, The Wilderness, and Health," Rogness pointed to this inner sacred space. During the presentation Rogness stated, "The goal of solitude and meditation is to take new levels of awareness into our daily life and situations. There is a direct connection between physiological well-being and emotional well-being. But mixed in there is an increased awareness of the spiritual sense of the Holy, the sacred, a deeper sense of peace and spiritual well-being." Many people, when they begin to listen to themselves, sense the Holy in their lives. Men universally talk about being called to move beyond themselves and into relationship with others and life after they have pulled away and gone into their solitude.

Neil Chethik shared the story about his father, who cried with him when his grandfather died. Chethik's father said, "I am crying not only for my father, but for me. His death means that I'll never hear the words I always wanted to hear from him: that he was proud of me, proud of the family I've raised and the life I've lived" (2001, 3).

Chethik was astounded when his father wept with him. Never before had he seen his father cry. Then his father gave Chethik a blessing – the one that he himself had not received. The father told his son how proud he was of him – for the life he was living and the family he was raising. Those words gave the son courage and confidence. Paradoxically, while honoring his son, the father was honoring his own father, who had not voiced such things to him. This became a sacred part of the relationship between Chethik and his father (2001).

Why Men Seek Solitude

When men enter their solitude, they let go of the external world. In so doing, they typically:

- Enter into an inner world that has its own noise that must be discerned.
- Work to hear more clearly the world they left.
- Often experience being loved.
- Figure out what they need for themselves.
- Figure out what to do for others.
- Learn from the memory of being loved about how to care for and to love others as they prepare to move beyond their inner solitude.
- Choose to move into relationship with others again.

In solitude, men work to sort out doing from being and give room to both. The purpose is to become more whole, and to find a balance between being separate and connected. We now look at three reasons why men seek solitude.

To Heal and Grow

As we have seen, solitude provides safety – a place where a man can tend to his wounds without being in harm's way. There he can entrust himself into the sacred space to sort through how to cope with what has happened and relate once again to others. One man who talked about the loss of his elderly mother said that family members were worried about their father after their mother died, fearing he would implode. "But we found out what he was made of and that it wasn't going to happen." His long life of coping with struggles and losses, as well as knowing he was loved, would serve him as he began to work through the loss of his wife.

Men seek solitude to know themselves and how to share or report their story. They also seek solitude to know how to relate to others. We often love people as we need them or as a child loves a parent. As we mature, we learn to truly love a parent by moving beyond the dependent way we need to love the parent. That involves moving beyond knowledge about another person to an appreciation of their life. Perhaps the way we do that is by coming to know one another's stories. What we learn from solitude is that we have to know our own story before we can share or report it.

To Be in Relationship

When we go within ourselves, we learn how to be with others. Men who have experienced depression report a difference between isolation and solitude. Solitude was not seen as the isolation, loneliness, or despair felt when in depression. The difference lies in how solitude teaches us to relate to ourselves *and* to move beyond ourselves. As we learn to relate to our own needs, we learn how to identify with and to reach out to others. One man saw how solitude was important, saying, "In solitude, I'm able to let go of demands and quietly get reconnected to self and what's important." By trusting solitude, he discovered what and who were important to him.

Both men and women need to learn to listen to each other more fully if they are going to learn what the other has to offer. They must love each other for who they *are* and not who they want each other to *be*. That involves respect, honor, integrity, and hard work.

To Find Wisdom
A man seeks solitude for healing, growth, relationship, and *wisdom*. Ibn Gabirol, poet and philosopher (c. 1022-1058), said, "In seeking wisdom, the first step is silence, the second listening, the third remembering, the fourth practicing, the fifth teaching others." It is interesting that Gabirol puts the sequence of steps in that order. He begins with silence, listening, and remembering. All of these are done in the inner self, although remembering can be shared.

Some people come to know that the Holy resides in solitude as the "still small voice" that quiets the soul. This quieting of the soul allows us to listen to that voice and to choose what needs to be heard. This is what some traditions call "soul work." As men learn to validate themselves, they learn how to do the same for others. As they experience being loved and validated by the Holy or what is meaningful to them, they learn how to love and validate others. For many men, solitude teaches this important lesson.

Solitude teaches us how to be wise in our relationships. Hebrew writings say that the beginning of wisdom is knowledge and that we know a wise person by what he or she does and the care they give. Wisdom, then, is using what we know in a loving way.

+ + +

It is important to recognize that when men seek solitude, they are not being passive or isolating themselves. It is just the opposite. Solitude is full of relational, life-giving, and healing work. Solitude teaches us to move toward our inner selves and to know ourselves, our strengths and weaknesses, and our joys and pains. Solitude teaches us to respect the need to know and relate to ourselves. We learn to value relationship by learning to relate to ourselves. Finally, solitude teaches us that we must choose to relate to others – to move beyond ourselves.

CHAPTER 7   THE ROLE OF THE WITNESS

I wrote the following song for Stan, who after many decades, began to revisit painful events of World War II that he had lived through.

"You Don't Have To Understand"

I just want my story to be heard.
You don't have to understand.
Just hear me out.
Let me know my words fall upon your soul.
Just hear me out,
I just want my words to fall upon some soul.

Today, I found myself needing a friend.
I touched upon a part of my life
I thought I'd left behind.
But it came, and I couldn't walk away this time.
So, I stayed there,
And, from it, this time, I really couldn't hide.

I felt the things I couldn't feel long ago.
The sorrow I could not bear,
Now, it breaks me down.
A war fought long ago
Comes back to haunt, now.
Hear my words, they're all I have to give you now.

He cried as he visited scene after scene.
It was as if his flowing tears
Fell on hallowed ground.
I listened as he shared from a wounded heart,

And I felt ashamed
I had not known what was on this man's heart.

So, I listened to my friend and his words,
And I came to know his heart
Though I couldn't understand.
But his words went deep into my soul.
I cried with him, too.
As his ancient tears fell upon my soul.

I just want my story to be heard.
You don't have to understand.
Just hear me out.
Let me know my words fall upon your soul.
Just hear me out,
I just want my words to fall upon some soul.

Daniel R. Duggan, Spring 2004

When men feel safe, when they have had a chance to sort through their thoughts, feelings, and what they want to do, they often come to a point where they want to be heard. Because men may need more time to process these things in their interior world, it may take them time to become ready to report on what happened to them and how they are coping.

That is also true for many men who faced the trauma of war. In 1994, the 50th anniversary of D-Day, the Allied landing on the beaches of Normandy, was celebrated. Thousands of U.S. World War II veterans made the trek back for the celebration. Younger Americans were in awe of their parents, grandparents, uncles, aunts, and friends who traveled back in time to find a way to remember, to honor, and (for many) to find closure, and 50 years later, tears fell for many as they remembered the horrors of war and their fallen comrades.

Stan's Stories

In the course of writing this book, I connected with an old friend, Stan. I had the opportunity to visit with him numerous times in which he shared stories about his life. Stan had grown up on a farm with immigrant parents. His father died early in the family's life. His mother remarried. Stan worked for farmers and at other labor jobs until he entered the war in 1941, at the age of 23. After serving stateside in the South and in the Northeast, he went to Ireland, where he was shipped to North Africa. He quickly encountered combat. He told stories of "how Rommel kicked our butts." When the campaign in North Africa was over, Stan moved with his troops to Italy. He spent three years overseas. During that time he faced some of the fiercest conflict and deprivation with little respite.

As we sat in his home some 60 years later, he reported vividly on men, events, names of villages and mountain passes, descriptions of tanks exploding and mortars bursting overhead, and details of equipment and artillery. Tears readily streamed down his face and mine as he quietly reported scenes of combat and tragedy. He said how real those memories still were and how long those three years felt. In his words, they "seemed like a lifetime." Stan never lost the memories. As we visited in his home, he did not talk much about his feelings – but his feelings were present in his words and storytelling.

He told me the story of his third Christmas during the war when he was finally furloughed for a home visit. He arrived in Chicago Christmas night, eager to surprise his three sisters. A taxi driver picked him up from the train station and took him to his sisters' boardinghouse. His sisters, however, were back in Iowa on the farm with their parents. Stan had to stay a block away that night in a room he could still describe with emotion – a tiny room with a pull-down bed with barely two feet around the edge for walking. Christmas night was spent alone. He had had no food the whole day. The hotel clerk had only two beers that he could give Stan for supper.

The next morning he walked to his sisters' boardinghouse and was let in by the woman who ran it. Because of the family resemblance, she knew he must be their brother. Their room was empty, but the refrigerator contained a pound of bacon and five eggs. He told me how he made himself the best-smelling breakfast he would ever remember. As he was fixing breakfast, his sisters walked in, having returned from Iowa. Stan's eyes were full of tears as he told the story. He took the train home to see his parents. After he arrived in his hometown, he received a ride to his family's farm from a fellow passenger who knew him and refused to let him go alone on this welcome home journey. This was the first time he had been home in three and a half years.

My visits often lasted two hours. I sat and listened. I could not understand the depth of his words or tears. I found myself in awe of a part of a man's life that was new to me, even though I had known him for 30 years. I knew he had been in the war, but I had no idea what he carried within himself all those years. Ruth, his wife, often left us alone but at the end of each visit was sincerely grateful when she said,

"Thank you for coming." I assured her it had been my pleasure. I should have said, "It has been my privilege."

A Time to Remember
Throughout our visits, Stan continued to talk about his war stories. As our visits progressed, we talked about our families and lives. The scope of our conversation broadened to include more of life. Five years previously, Stan had shared a war story with his wife for the first time. This seemed to open the door for more conversations with family members and confidants. In these revelations, Stan was finally able to report these stories in the depth of his feelings. This was often more than he had experienced when old war friends gathered for reunions.

Stan had some thoughts about why this was so for him. First, when he returned home from the war, men talked about where they had been and so on. But in his view, they were also endeavoring to get on with the rest of their lives. Like Stan, they quickly entered the workforce, began families, and strove to make the best of their sacrifice. It doesn't surprise me that we had such an economic boom following the war. So many people were pulling together for the same reason. Stan was one of those people.

One thing he observed about himself was that while he worked long and hard hours during the week, he also needed to keep busy on the weekends; otherwise, he wound up with downtime to remember. As he aged, he could not be as active. With time on his hands, he was forced to think and remember. He was not surprised when he started talking about his war memories when he was 75.

It could be said that Stan spent a lifetime in his cave isolating himself from his memories and feelings about the war by fulfilling his role as provider. As he aged and had time to think back on his life, he revisited old memories. Healing began when he was able to report his memories and have them heard and witnessed. He reconnected to the part of himself that he had spent a lifetime disassociating from. He was beginning to find doors that allowed him to journey into his core of grief.

How the Witness Honors

It was an honor to be with Stan. I always felt like I was on holy ground when he shared his stories and his life.

Stan was a good teacher, reminding me how to be with a man in his grief. I was lucky enough to know to follow his lead. I knew that I was invited into the sacred space of his stories and feelings. That called me to be present with my heart. I was also called to witness the report. Stan reported what had happened. His words were incredibly fresh and clear as if the events had just happened.

Sometimes a story needs to be told several times or in several ways before it feels finished. That was not the case with Stan. As I listened, I sensed that a soldier was reporting on his mission. Through these stories, this old soldier permitted himself to now report on how much terror and loss he had seen and experienced. For this work, he needed me simply to be a witness.

While listening, I realized that Stan did not need me to interrupt him by asking questions, sharing my feelings or thoughts, or interjecting something of my own. What he needed was a quiet presence. I felt like a sponge soaking up his stories. That was my only task. Sometimes it was hard to just sit and listen. I had been trained to interact verbally with the other person. I never stopped being in awe of how profound an experience it was to be present to Stan and his journey. What I realized was how both of us were connecting and developing rapport emotionally.

Finally, Stan taught me about the nature of men's tears. Stan's tears came easily. Perhaps some of that could be attributed to his age, when tears may come more easily. But he also had many tears stored away. The important lesson about tears is that they do not always have to be addressed. Stan's tears came from what he was talking about. They were doing their work. I never felt the need to ask Stan about them. I chose to remain quiet and simply listen, reverently, to what they pointed to in his words. He wanted his words to be heard. He did not need to be understood. He simply wanted his story to be witnessed. My quiet presence was the witness that validated his being heard and honored him.

During one of our visits, I sang to Stan "You Don't Have to Understand," the song I had written from my experience of being with him. At the end of the song, I thanked him for the sacrifice he had made for me during the war.

How the Witness Is Engaged

The witness is not just a bystander or passive listener. The witness is employing respect and honor. Witnessing is what rapport is about when men are talking respectfully to one another. By listening respectfully, even without the necessity to understand everything, two people enter into a bond of trust and mutual respect. The speaker, not having to explain the meaning of everything, is satisfied that he has been heard. Hearing means receiving the speaker as well as the message. This is validation. This is what is important to a man who needs to tell his story.

We all want to be heard, but the needs that are met may be different. A woman may wish to be heard in a way that she is understood by the other. A man may need to know that his words are heard but simply in a way that another has witnessed his story. He may not feel the need to be understood fully. If he is fully understood, he might feel a loss of some of his independence and autonomy. He might become like others and less of his unique self. Respecting differences honors the nature and mystery of the journey to healing and wholeness.

In a workshop on men and grief, Joseph Kilikevich (2000) said, "When you are finished telling the story, you are finished with the story." Men need to have a witness, so the story can be finished and the grief let go.

+ + +

In having a story witnessed, a man no longer feels alone or isolated with his grief or pain. The witness plays an important role in healing. Witnessing is a quiet presence that remains long after the experience and is remembered within. Such an experience teaches us about the importance of reaching out and moving beyond ourselves.

CHAPTER 8   HOW TO HELP MEN IN GRIEF

"What Am I Going to Do Without Mama" or "When Anger Looks Our Way"

A 73-year-old woman died in the hospital with her family by her side. She had a long history of complicated medical problems but, according to family members, had always "bounced back."

The woman died before I arrived on the floor. I went to her room and spent a moment of silence and prayer with her. Then, I met the family in the waiting room: the husband, a son, a daughter, and a sister-in-law, along with some friends. The son and daughter were sitting on either side of their father talking with and comforting him while he exclaimed, "What am I going to do without Mama?" They did not seem to know how to respond to their father. They attempted to assuage his feelings by quickly reassuring him that they would be there for him. Their attempts, however, did not seem to work.

Soon they began telling stories. I stood quietly as it appeared they were doing what they needed to be doing. The storytelling flowed between all the family and friends. Eventually, grief overwhelmed the husband again. He expressed anger at why this had to happen to his wife. He had expected that she would rebound as before. He became frustrated when the doctors told him why they thought she had died. When they returned a second time to discuss it with him, he became angry and upset.

Again, his children became anxious. They attempted to tell him why he should not feel this way, saying, "Mom was worn out, Dad. The doctors and nurses did all they could." It was then that I approached him and knelt down and said, "I don't know how you must be feeling right now. It must be awful. I believe you have a right to feel whatever you're feeling. I want you to know that." I then asked, "Is there anything I can do to help you with what you are angry about?" At that point, all in the room were watching us. He paused and said, "I don't think so. I'm just so upset. I don't know what to do." I said, "I think we can all understand that." Two or three minutes of silence followed. Finally, he said, "Thank you."

From that point on, he was able to move into his own storytelling. He was able to give space to his daughter's and son's feelings and wanted to hear what they had to say. At times, they'd cry together over a story or memory. When they were ready to go into the woman's room, they were supportive of one another. After the family had time for telling stories, holding her hand, and spending quiet time with her, I offered a prayer. About five minutes later, I excused myself to give them some alone time as a family.

When I returned, they were leaving the room. The son hung back, so I stayed with him. "This must be a very hard thing," I said.

He agreed saying, "She's always been a wonderful mother. I knew this would happen someday, but I never realized what it would be like."

"Your heart is pretty sad," I replied. "I'm sad for you, too. I'm glad you were here with her, your dad, and sister."

The son reported, "My brother is still flying in from the coast."

"Gee, I'm sorry. I can imagine that it would have meant a lot to you to have him here with you," I added.

He nodded and cried while I embraced him. He talked some more about the day and what had happened. He was soon ready to leave and join the rest of the family.

+ + +

We can identify several doors into grief the family used in the above story. The first is that until the husband's *anger* was heard and accepted – *witnessed* – he seemed to be unduly troubled by the situation. It felt like he was at the door of his grief and needed to enter but was not being permitted to do so.

Anger is an important element of grief. When anger is misunderstood or shut down, it can impede grieving and healing. Acknowledging the husband's anger was an important moment for him and for the family. It gave him permission to feel his anger with someone who could hear it and not try to take it away. It gave his children permission to accept where he was in his grief. This helped him to deal with other feelings associated with his loss and enabled the family to work through a tough spot in their grief work. Behind his anger lay feelings of helplessness and panic as he tried to cope with and make sense of the shock he was feeling. *Anger* and *panic* became doors for the husband to enter more fully into his grief. He needed a safe place for that to happen.

The husband and other family members were at different places along *the continuum of grief work*. This confused the family members because they did not know how to respond to their father's anger and be supportive of him in the way that he needed. There can be many reasons for these differences within a family such as depth of relationship or closeness, roles, timing, personality, suddenness versus long-term suffering, and so on.

We could also wonder if the children's discomfort was connected to seeing the helplessness of their father, as expressed in his words: "What am I going to do without Mama?" Children can feel anxious, no matter how old they are, when their parents express vulnerability. That may be even truer *when the parent is a father and is expressing his vulnerability through emotions and panic.* In this case, the children responded by care-taking rather than simply witnessing his feelings. This can be broadened to many situations when men express themselves emotionally in a crisis or loss. The male's emotional expressions can elicit an emotional distancing of others and a stance of care-taking, judging, and/or avoidance. It is as if the people around them do not know how to be present to the emotionally expressive male, or, as one of my colleagues noted, the family in this story might have felt shock at seeing an emotion never expressed before by their father.

Again, we see the role of *storytelling* in this instance. We need to recognize that storytelling normally does not occur until the shock of death begins to subside and some of the feelings and thoughts begin to be available to the individual. The husband could not be denied his feelings. I suspect that his panic may well have been associated with his fear that his anger would not be heard and accepted. If anger is one of the few feelings males are permitted to have in our culture, then being denied his anger meant being denied his grief, too. He innately knew that his anger was the key to his sorrow. He needed to have his anger honored and respected.

Then he could enter more fully into the deeper purpose of storytelling, which is to connect one to the greater range of feelings that loss engenders.

Another characteristic of this story that shows how grief is expressed is *relationship*. Relationship was a door that each of the family members (including the husband) used to enter their grief. They used their relationships with one another, their loved one who had died, the chaplain, others not present, and God to help them give expression to their sorrow and grief work.

What is interesting is *when* the individuals selected this door of relationship. The husband wanted his anger to be witnessed before he could enter deeper into relationship with family members. The son chose to go into his *cave* and invited the chaplain to be there with him as he reported what was important to him. Note that I used feeling words and empathy to connect with him, but the son did what he needed to do and reported what was going on in his inner world. If we were to intuit his feelings, his words dripped with emotion. He was doing the work that he needed to do.

Lastly, there was a reason I dismissed myself from the family. Just as an individual may need to be alone, a family may need room for *solitude* from the world – a place where they can tend to their wounds, find inner strength, and gain the wisdom to face their broken world.

Much of what I present in this book runs counter to what has been taught in Western culture. Most of us were not trained to see solitude as a positive response to grief or storytelling as a way for men to express feelings. We were not trained to appreciate that a man may not have to name and express feelings as his first step into the core of grief. The challenge for those who help grieving men is not only to learn new skills, but also to be willing to learn about ourselves and move beyond our own comfort zones. The following is meant as a way to begin as you walk with men through grief.

Ways to Help Men in Grief

1. Create safe places.
2. Be realistic.
3. Be a witness.
4. Trust solitude and its work.
5. Help restore self-esteem.
6. Support the family system.
7. Invite ways for men to do things in their grief work.
8. Accept anger.
9. Think differently about how a man expresses feelings.
10. Know the importance of story.
11. Recognize the importance of honor and respect.

Create Safe Places

Our role when caring for a man in grief is to help create safe relationships and spaces in which he can do what he needs to do for himself. If a man does not feel safe, he will not entrust another with his stories or feelings. We all need to feel accepted for who we are and for our way of coping. We all know what it feels like when we are not accepted or when we feel like someone is trying to direct us in a way that makes the other person feel better. Safety is the starting point for helping others.

You do not have to remake yourself in order to create safe relationships and places for others who are different from you. In other words, you do not have to be like another person or understand another person for that person to feel safe with you. Acceptance of others for who they are is key. Know what their grieving preference looks like and be willing to respond with acceptance even when it may not feel or seem natural to you. In helping relationships, men have had to learn to be sensitive to a feminine style of being and coping. Now women have to learn how to be sensitive to a masculine style of coping, or men will not feel safe to share or report their story.

Be willing to be a safe person to men. Value solitude. Know that it is deep and intrinsic to many men as they cope with life. Practice gender wholeness. When you see some men expressing their "feminine side," accept it for what it is. A man may be uncomfortable with it or see it as feminizing. The beginning of diversity in grief is safety.

Do not rush to help men in grief if you are not willing, able, or capable of being present with them on their own terms. They will see through your façade and turn away. If you are unsure about how to be helpful, trust that most men appreciate being asked what would be helpful. Then follow their suggestions.

Finally, do not be afraid to step back and get out of the way if the man and his family are doing what they need to be doing for themselves.

Be Realistic

Ask yourself: "What can I realistically hope to accomplish?" You cannot do the work for a man. He has to go through the door that leads to the core of grief for himself. You cannot force him, and you need to be accepting when he does not do what you think might be helpful to him. Alcoholics Anonymous teaches, "Let go and let God" – meaning that we cannot manage other people.

Be mindful of your agenda. Each man is a unique individual with his own experiences and style of coping. I have seen some people eager to help. In their eagerness, they become impatient and forget to follow the lead of the person whom they are trying to support. Such enthusiasm can have the effect of making the other person feel unsafe.

Be a Witness

This is one of those areas that can feel counter-intuitive when working with men and their grief because it may seem like there is a need to ask questions for clarification or inquire about feelings. However, this only interrupts the man and keeps him from telling his story.

Witness the story. Do not interrupt when listening. Remember that you do not have to say anything. Many times men simply want their stories heard, as we saw with Stan in chapter 7. Men may not need to be understood, but they most often need or want to be heard. It is validating to the one who is grieving to know that his story has been heard. In the end say, "Thank you for telling me your story."

Allow for silence as a part of a man's storytelling or reporting. It is not unusual for a man to use long periods of silence as a way to collect his thoughts before knowing how to frame a story or choose what to report on. Tom Golden (2001) makes the point that when counseling, he has often waited five to seven minutes for a man to respond. In doing so, he sensed how the man was often thinking through what he wanted to say and how he wanted to say it. Being present while a man is thinking is also a way to witness. Men may use fewer words, as well. Golden notes that research has shown that women may use 7,000 words daily to express themselves; men may use 2,000.

Trust Solitude and Its Work

If we are truly going to be helpful to men, we must value solitude. Men learn about relating to themselves, others, life, and the Holy as they enter their solitude. When a man experiences a loss, he often moves into solitude. There he attends to his wounds, sorts through what has happened, deals with feelings, trusts the self and others who are there with him, and learns how he wants to move beyond the cave and into the world of external relationships again.

Trust solitude. When a man needs to be alone to deal with what has happened, important healing work may be going on. By being comfortable with the man's need for space, we are showing that we trust his ability to know what he needs to do for himself. More importantly, we are showing respect for him, which enables him to build a strong bridge between us.

Help Restore Self-Esteem

While self-esteem often grows for the female through emotional relationships, the male's preference may be through autonomy and doing. Recognize that a loss may have struck a blow to a male's self-esteem because he could not protect or prevent the loss. The rush of feelings may be more than he can handle, causing him to feel overwhelmed.

Here again, accepting and respecting the man's need for solitude while he collects himself is a way to help him restore his self-esteem. Self-esteem comes to us when we are doing what we need to do for ourselves. When a man moves into his solitude, he learns to use his own inner strength to deal with life.

One anxious young father was given the task of keeping a cool washcloth upon his child's feverish forehead. In doing this, he found a way to express his tenderness, which seemed to alleviate some of his fears. This allowed him to connect with his child and to find other ways to be present to his child and family.

Support the Family System

Give support, affirmation, and safe space to the family system. Work to provide a safe space for family members to cope with their loss in their own unique ways. Then step back and get out of the way. The family system will often rise to the occasion and do what only it can do for itself, using both feminine and masculine gender characteristics to help them cope.

Recognize and affirm a male's place in the family. Do not dismiss, slight, minimize, or judge him when he and his loved ones are experiencing a loss. Men are often viewed in negative ways when they are misunderstood or not accepted. Destructive or harmful behavior cannot be tolerated. Yet, we need to recognize that our judgments and biases are not helpful.

Invite Ways for Men to Do Things in Their Grief Work

Value "doing" as a way of expressing emotions. Men use doing as a way of working through their grief. Help men to think about ways they can do things to give meaning to their loss and grief. Ask what they have been thinking they could do. Learn to pursue together what works for them. Do not assume that because men are less demonstrative with their feelings they lack a need to express their grief. Invite men to do things that serve and nurture others. As a starting point, ask the man to tell you what happened or how he reacted.

You can help men find rituals that help them express their grief through doing something important that has meaning and gives honor. I have often encouraged a man to write a letter and read it at the cemetery. Some men build something or plant a tree in the yard to honor or express their feelings. In the Jewish tradition, loved ones who have died are often named during special family occasions or religious rituals as a way to remember them. In time, the family members begin to see the progress they have made in their journey with grief. Rituals enable them to find new meanings.

Accept Anger

Do not assume that when a man shares anger with you that it is about you. It may be more about feeling unsafe or feeling too vulnerable. Let him have his feeling of anger. You may be the only anchor that he has against harming himself or someone else. If you are concerned, let him know what the limits are, but acknowledge that you hear his pain. Ask him if there is anything you can do to help him with his anger.

Remember, you are not responsible for his anger. Anger is a secondary feeling in that it is connected to another feeling the individual is experiencing such as hurt or fear; anger is the only way he has to express it. In our culture, anger is one of the few feelings men are permitted. The primary feeling underneath the anger is normally not as acceptable for men. If you take away or do not acknowledge the anger, you may be shutting the only door he has to enter into his core of grief.

Think Differently About How a Man Expresses Feelings

Do not assume that a man does not have feelings simply because you cannot see them. Most likely, he has taken them into his cave where he is trying to express, name, cope, and find meaning. Then he has to choose how he will move beyond his cave and socialize his grief in a way that is meaningful to him while helping others dealing with the loss, too.

Remember that men often get to their feelings, but the naming and expression of feelings may come at the end of their grief work rather than at the beginning. What is noteworthy is that if men do not find a safe place to step into their core of grief and pass through it to the other side, grief may become long-term, unresolved grief. Each man has to find the door that is natural and safe for him.

How can we help men deal with feelings? Avoid asking, "How are you feeling?" – at least until you sense that he has words for his feelings. Instead ask, "How are you doing?" Additionally, assist men in finding ways to do things in their grief work, such as making phone calls or arrangements, or building something symbolic. Feelings are often expressed in doing meaningful things. Provide openers for storytelling such as, "What happened?" or "How did you hear about it?" Give them space to go into their emotional cave. Do not blame or become resentful when they do so. Trust that their silence may be sacred to them since solitude has great strength in it. When they begin to tell their story, listen quietly without interrupting.

Know that men's grief sometimes triggers feelings of helplessness. It is common to feel caught off guard and surprised by a man who is weeping. You may feel that the man is weak and undisciplined, despite your best intentions. You may be shocked by how quickly negative feelings arise. Those feelings may have deep roots in your psyche. Being aware of such thoughts or feelings can enable you to ask yourself, "What does this man in grief need from me?"

Know the Importance of Story

Men eventually get to feelings once they have entered their grief and begin telling their stories. Again, once a story is told, the grief work may be done. In other words, the feelings were expressed in the telling of the story. This may be all that is necessary for now. It is like peeling the proverbial onion. Healing takes place when one is ready to peel away that layer.

Multiple doors may be involved. The door a man enters that allows him to peel one layer may be different from the next one, until he finishes peeling away all the layers of sorrow that are there. For some, that work is never finished. If you are in doubt about whether or not the story is completed, ask something like, "Is there more?" or "Do you feel done?" Trust the obvious.

Recognize the Importance of Honor and Respect

Help men to have honor in their grief. Death often confronts men with a sense of failure because they feel they have not ultimately protected their families. Honor them by giving them space to go into their caves without being judged. Trust that their silence may be sacred to them. Trust their anger and the other feelings that help open the doors of grief. Honor their loss.

Encourage men to do their best. If you sense someone is feeling helpless, you might ask, "What is going to be the most helpful thing for your family or friends?" Let them hear they are okay, loved, and accepted. Speak their names aloud in prayer or conversation. Listen quietly when they begin to tell their story. Doing so honors their sharing.

Tom Golden reported on one prerequisite for men to share their grief that is related to the issue of hierarchy. Golden wrote, "For a man to share his grief he needs to know that he is respected" (2000, 80). Respect is related to hierarchy. A man often does not want to burden someone with his grief if that person has no responsibility for it. If a man chooses not to share his grief with you, respect his choice.

Many men will stand in the face of great pain, threat, and even death to do what is honorable. It is an important part of their identity, as it harkens back to the roots of their gender identity in the roles of provider and protector. When they can find honor in doing what they are called to do for their families, friends, and larger communities, they enter into actions that are healing for them.

+ + +

Finally, remember men may expect women to move beyond their need to have sadness and grief surface in relationships before they are ready to do so. Women, in turn, may expect men to move beyond solitude and into relationships before they are ready to do so. My encouragement is to understand differences and to bless the many natural ways of healing rather than assuming there is only one way.

Openness to possible gender differences in grieving styles allows us to learn from one another, to do some healing between the genders, to enable healthy differentiation, and to bless our uniqueness and commonalities with one another.

CHAPTER 9   WHEN YOU ARE THE MAN WHO IS GRIEVING

We all must go through the "core of grief" in order to heal. Every important loss in our lives leaves a mark upon us. Some stand out and cause us to have to rework how we cope with loss – sometimes with life itself. When the wound of grief is unattended or not channeled into something positive, the energy generated by the loss does not go away. It can transform into either depression or patterns of feelings including anger, resentment, blame, self-pity, or guilt.

If we do not deal with the grief of sorrow, we are left with the grief of regrets. Our soul, spirit, or psyche knows when we have not attended to our inner work. Healing begins when we do and say what we need to do and say. If what we need to attend to is our sorrow, then we need to give ourselves permission to be sad and grieve.

Don't Assume All Grief Is the Same

A word of caution: Although many men may experience a significant loss, they may find that what they learned about grief and coping does not seem to help them when they experience an even greater loss. They may have to learn to walk through a new door or go back and deal with a new level of an earlier grief.

To illustrate, my father's abandonment had always been the great loss in my life. That loss defined me in some ways. I developed some strengths because of it. But it was not until my late 30s when I lost, as the result of a merger, a department I had started that I could begin to deal with the loss of my father more completely. This department had been almost like a child to me. I started the department, watched it grow, attended to it, and felt like a proud "father." Then, the "child" was taken. I had no recourse. Everything I had learned about grief and coping no longer worked for me. I went into a tailspin and struggled to pull out of it.

I knew that my behaviors and feelings were becoming dangerous to my career. My anger was on the surface most of the time. I was full of resentment and self-pity. It would not go away. I felt helpless and unsure of myself. Some of my professional relationships were deteriorating. My relationships with family and friends were being affected, too.

This experience of loss was completely new to me. I did not know how to cope. I knew I needed help. By the time I started looking for help, a part of me had gone deep into my cave. Surprisingly, it was there that I noticed my feelings of loss and sorrow for my father.

Ten years earlier, I used counseling to deal with some of the rage and anger I had toward my father for abandoning us. While that counseling had helped me deal with rage and anger, it had not helped me work through the sorrow I felt about his absence. I believed that those feelings of sorrow held a clue that would help me deal with the loss of the department and what that loss meant to me. I entered into grief counseling again. It was the first time that I was able to name feelings of sorrow for the father I had and the father I wished I'd had. I found a peace with my father that I had not known before.

I learned about the importance of working through the great losses in my life. I learned that doing this work helped prepare me for the great losses to come. It was not until I worked through the core of grief with my father's abandonment that I could face the loss of my department with greater acceptance and resolution. In retrospect, part of my helplessness in dealing with the loss of my department was connected to a myth. I thought that I should have known what I needed to know to help me deal with this new loss and challenge. That was a myth.

What is the lesson in all of this? Do not assume you know what you need to know about how to cope with loss. Each new loss may have something to teach you about the past, the present, and the future.

Choose to Risk Vulnerability (or Choose What YOU Want to Live For)

When we were boys, we often played games of competition, conflict, and war. Each time we played those games, we were rehearsing anthropological roles for which nature was preparing us. We were learning about the warrior/protector and provider roles. In these games of boyhood, we were learning about sacrificing ourselves.

In adulthood, we have to discover what we want to live for. We men may find it easy to live out our roles as protector and provider. Those roles are important dimensions of our living within families and the many communities of which we are a part. A trait of many men is that we will put ourselves in harm's way or sacrifice ourselves to honor our commitment to family and provide for their well-being. We are wired that way.

But it seems that we are not wired as well to deal with the many emotions that arise in relationships and in grief.

Sometimes we may try to permanently escape our feelings by burying ourselves in busyness or work. When we do this, however, we are not honoring relationships or the ones we loved. To heal from the wounds of grief, we have to risk leaning into our vulnerability and feelings. Honoring our vulnerability allows us to stand on sacred ground. As the biblical writer Paul wrote, "When I am weak, I am strong." (II Corinthians 12:10 RSV).

To help us deal with feelings, we may even need to learn new skills, such as naming feelings, doing something with them, or talking about them. The issue is choosing what we are going to face in order to live. We have to choose to enter our core of grief so we can heal in our relationships and from our grief. This is a choice to live through the pain and find new hope. It is a choice to risk vulnerability in order to live.

Know How Your Anger Is Affecting Others

It is paradoxical, but anger is one of the few feelings that our culture allows men to name and express. Men can often name anger before we can name other feelings. It is also a feeling that gets men into trouble when it is unbridled. In previous generations, men could find places and male relationships where they could be mentored in dealing with their roles, the challenges of life, and relationships. Today that is often not so. Modern men may not get the necessary input and feedback about the need to modulate anger and when to do so.

Many men are surprised by how others experience their expression of anger. They often share that their anger is simply an emotional expression meant to vent. They are not prepared to hear that those who are the recipients of their anger feel shut down, abused, and afraid. Even in grief, a man's anger can be intimidating to others. So the one feeling he knows the most about can also create distress, loss, and isolation when he is attempting just the opposite.

Grief involves many feelings. At times, grief can feel crazy. Anger is commonly the first feeling many men use to give expression to what has happened to them. Often men are trying to work through other feelings when anger comes out, but the anger is typically the only expression available to them on an emotional level. It is here that a man's anger is often misunderstood.

As we've seen, anger is typically a secondary feeling that masks another feeling underneath. Men have to learn to recognize the feeling beneath the anger, to name it, and to give it appropriate expression. While feelings may not be our strength, we *are* wired to have them. It may simply take us longer to get to them. We may have to get to them from another direction. Doing something meaningful or finding solitude where we get in touch with feelings, such as sorrow, can help us move beyond ourselves and share our grief. In any case, anger is often a clue that we are hurting about something. If we are going to deal with our grief, we need to acknowledge our anger, move beyond it, and deal with the hurt. (Remember the husband who became angry at his children for minimizing his fear of how he would live without his wife.)

We do not have the right to take our anger out on another person. That is what gets many men – and women – in trouble. Anger that turns into physical violence or emotional abuse is never acceptable. If you have a pattern in which anger moves into rage, physical violence, or emotional abuse, then that is a sign you need to find help to look beneath the anger and see what feelings and memories are attached to it. You may find such help in a men's meeting or group where it is safe to talk about oneself, with a male mentor, or through counseling from a clergyperson or counselor. It is okay to ask for help and seek meaningful male friendships.

As men, we need to learn to help each other when we see family members or friends getting out of control. For example, you might ask, "Hey, what is your anger about?" or "What is so upsetting?" or simply say, "You seem upset." We also need to be willing to let each other know that violent behavior is not acceptable. Such anger is not only hurting someone else, it prevents us from effectively dealing with the issue that we need to deal with.

We need to recognize how our anger is affecting others. We need to be sensitive to how we express anger so that it does not overwhelm the other person. It might be helpful to let the other person know that you are angry or upset about something and to ask to talk about it. Form an agreement with the other person that you will share your anger, that you are willing to hear his or her feelings or response, and that you are open to feedback.

In all fairness, many men possess a wide range of feelings, and they name and give them expression in appropriate ways. Anger may not need to play such a pivotal role in the expression of feelings. In general, we need to learn to name a wider range of feelings within us. When we name what needs addressing, we also find ways to deal with it. As the old adage says, "We can deal with what we know. We cannot deal with what we do not know."

Trust Your Need for Solitude and When to Move Beyond It

Trust your need for solitude. Trust it and let it be your friend. Name what you need to name in your solitude. Find comfort in being present with yourself, memories, and conversations in solitude. Remember that one of the purposes of solitude is to teach you to relate to others, life, the Holy, or whatever you hold as good. Sometimes you need to go away and feel your pain and even the isolation that may come with it. That is a necessary part of healing for you to experience the loss that has entered your life.

However, when isolation begins to feel like a permanent state, you need to invite someone into your cave or choose to move beyond your isolation back into relationships. This can help you reconnect to your feelings of sorrow. If having crawled into your cave has turned into weeks or months or even years, you should consider either moving out into the world again or getting some help to move from isolation to solitude. Choosing *what* we will live for takes on new meaning when we again take the risk to invest our energies in relationships. Grief does not have to have the last word.

My own experience related to the death of my maternal grandmother when I was about 30 is a case in point. I was very close to her. She had asked me to officiate her funeral. Emotionally, family funerals were just too difficult for me, and I had told myself I would not do another one. However, I chose to officiate her funeral because I wanted to honor Grandma's request. What I did not realize was that I had put some of my grief on the back burner. Within a few weeks of returning to work, I realized I was experiencing some mild, lingering depression. I was beginning to feel isolated even from parts of myself. In the past, I would have moved on without giving it much more consideration.

However, at this point I knew enough to ask myself why I was feeling cut off and depressed. Initially, I was not sure why. Taking stock of what I had recently experienced helped me see my loss again. It was then that I got in touch with sorrow and feelings about Grandma's death. My way of handling my grief, in that moment, was to kneel and ask God to take care of Grandma now that we could no longer take care of her. I asked God to convey to her what I wanted to tell her. Then, in my prayer, I told Grandma what I wanted to tell her. This was my way of pouring out some of my sorrow and moving through my core of grief.

This grief work had to be intentional because my learned way of coping with grief was to avoid pain by getting busy and moving away from it, which was not healthy for me. In fact, that is why, in part, I was depressed when I went back to work. I realized that my energies were being spent avoiding grief rather than reaching out to life and relationships. For me, reaching out to someone in my solitude enabled me to express sorrow in my way and, eventually, share my feelings of sorrow with others. I was choosing to live again rather than spend my energies avoiding my core of grief, an important part of myself.

Know When to Separate Intimacy and Sex

Many books have been written on this topic. In our culture, intimacy for men is often connected to sex and romantic relationships. At a time when men may be ready for and need intimacy, as in grief, intimacy can be a problem if it is connected, in our minds, with sex. In grief, when we are ready to invite someone into our cave or to move beyond it, we need to separate our need for intimacy and our need for sex. That can help us be open to healing relationships around us.

We have all known men who lost a spouse and quickly became involved with another person to quell the loneliness and grief. Those new relationships were often short-lived. I have known men who remarried before working through their grief and who died within a year.

Be Open to Witness Another's Story

When other men share their grief, open yourself to be a witness. Be willing to ask, "What happened?" Let the other person know that it is okay with you to hear his story. Do not interrupt. Honor them by simply listening. Be patient and wait if needed. You are on holy ground when you are listening to another person share his grief. Be willing to be a witness. It is a gift that will not be forgotten.

Give Yourself Permission to Have Male Friendships

Friendships can be key in helping to get through tough times. But many of us do not have deep male friendships. We get caught up being providers or simply get caught in myths about individuality or competitiveness. We, men, can fear getting close. Whatever the reason, we wind up cutting ourselves off from relationships with other men who can befriend or mentor us when we most need it. Friendships can deepen your sense of yourself, others, and life.

Sometimes we have to give ourselves permission to develop friendships that are more than acquaintances or superficial relationships. I, for one, have had to learn to give myself permission to have friendships with men. I learned as a young man that I needed male friendships. As I got busy in my career, I did not feel like I had the time for friendships. Friendships were a luxury. However, I found that I could not be a husband, father, worker, and provider without rubbing shoulders with other men in friendships. So, at certain periods of my life, I was intentional in developing deeper relationships with men that enriched me as a man.

When I changed jobs in my early 40s, it took me five years before I began to acknowledge my need to develop new male friendships in my new community. I had maintained some old friendships from earlier in my life, but I had not given myself permission to develop new ones.

I discovered that I needed to change my attitude. I did this by helping to start a "Breakfast Club" of four men who meet once a month to talk about what is happening in our lives. I am also one of four men who helped to start two men's meetings called "I AM" that meet twice a month to simply listen to one another's stories without interruption and to dialogue about what is important to each other. This group began in the year 2000 and continues to meet with many of the same men. Before moving from that community, I met a friend about once a month for breakfast to catch up. During the spring and summer, I spend three weeks fishing and sharing camaraderie with friends and family at a resort in northern Minnesota. These are ways that I feed my male spirit.

We find friendship, camaraderie, and male bonding in many ways. When we find these kinds of relationships, they are bound to grow as we nurture them. We become better sons, husbands/lovers, fathers, uncles, cousins, and friends because other men know our stories. From such experiences, we learn how to listen and stand on sacred ground with others – men and women.

+ + +

We must learn to distinguish between isolation and solitude if we are going to move through the passages of our lives. This involves dealing with the great losses we encounter on our journey and healing from them. But we also may need to know that we do not have to be lone rangers or lone soldiers on our watch.

We need to learn to trust our solitude and what it has to give us. We need to hear when solitude calls us to move beyond ourselves, even with our grief. But we need others who can understand our way of being. Once we have been loved and honored for who we are, we need to give back what was given to us in our time of need.

I like to think that we stand at a crossroads in the course of history for men. We face a challenge to heal from many wounds, including grief. But we also face the challenge to learn how to be healers and to be creative in bringing what is unique about us as men to our families, friends, communities, culture, and world. In doing so, we are all made more whole.

I now work in a continuing care retirement center with elders. What they are teaching me is that life is full of change and loss. When we face change and loss, we have to decide what we are going to hang on to and what we are going to let go of as we deal with the things leaving us. We also have to deal with our losses. We deal with all of that by *expressing*, in our own way, what needs to be expressed, *naming* what needs to be named, *coping* with what we have named, and finding *meaning* in it. Part of our legacy is giving back by teaching others to walk through the doors of grief that fit them. As we have seen, one of those doors is the door of solitude. When we walk through it, we take its gift and find our way into life with others again.

REFERENCES

Anderson, Ray S. 1995. *Unspoken Wisdom – Truths My Father Taught Me.* Minneapolis: Augsburg.

Blauner, Bob. 1997. *Our Mothers' Spirits – On the Death of Mothers and the Grief of Men.* New York: Regan Books.

Bly, Robert. 1990. *Iron John.* Reading, MA: Addison.

Campbell, Joseph. 1976. *The Portable Jung.* New York: Penguin Books.

Chethik, Neil. 2000. "Reaching Bereaved Men Requires Innovation." *The Forum,* September/October.

Chethik, Neil. 2001. *FatherLoss – How Sons of All Ages Come to Terms with the Deaths of their Dads.* New York: Hyperion.

Doka, Kenneth. 1989. *Disenfranchised Grief: Recognizing Hidden Sorrow.* Lexington, MA: Lexington Press.

Doka, Kenneth, and Terry Martin. 2000. *Men Don't Cry...Women Do: Transcending Gender Stereotypes of Grief.* Bristol, PA: Taylor & Francis.

Gilligan, Carol, 1982. *In a Different Voice – Psychological Theory and Women's Development.* Cambridge: Harvard University Press.

Goebel, Julie. 1994. "Grief Experience Inventory." *GEI Review,* November, 4 (2).

Golden, Thomas R. 2000. *Swallowed by a Snake – The Gift of the Masculine Side of Healing.* Gaithersburg, MD: Golden Healing Publishing L.L.C.

Golden, Thomas R. 2001. "The Gift of the Masculine Side of Healing." Presented at the International Bereavement Conference On Death and Bereavement, Kings College. London, Ontario.

Heim, P., and S. Golant. 1992. *Hardball for Women: Winning at the Game of Business*. Los Angeles: Lowell House.

Keating, Thomas. 2003. "Spirituality and Health." Plenary Session. Association of Professional Chaplains National Convention.

Keen, Sam. 1992. *Fire in the Belly – On Being a Man*. New York: Bantam Books.

Kilikevich, Joseph. 2000. "How Do Men Grieve." Presented at the International Bereavement Conference On Death and Bereavement, Kings College. London, Ontario.

Moore, John H. 1989. *But What About Men – After Women's Lib*. Bath, Great Britain: Ashgrove Press Limited.

Moss, Miriam S., Sidney Z. Moss, and R. L. Rubinstein. 1996-97. "Middle-Aged Son's Reactions to Father's Death," *Omega* 34 (4): 259-277.

Rando, Therese. 1986. *Parental Loss of a Child*. Champaign, IL: Research Press Company.

Rogness, Andrew. 1994. *Crossing Boundary Waters*. Minneapolis: Augsburg.

Rogness, Andrew. 2006. "Solitude, The Wilderness, And Health." Medico-Clergy Conference, Gundersen Lutheran Medical Center, 2006.

Rosenblatt, P. C., R. P. Walsh, and D. A. Jackson. 1976. *Grief and Mourning in Cross-Cultural Perspective*. H.R.A.F. Press.

Somé, Malidoma Patrice. 1993. *Ritual: Power, Healing and Community*. Portland: Swan Raven and Company.

Staudacher, Carol. 1989. *Beyond Grief: A Guide for Recovering from the Death of a Loved One*. Oakland: New Harbinger Publications, Inc.

Staudacher, Carol. 1991. *Men and Grief*. Oakland: New Harbinger Publications, Inc.

Viorst, Judith. 1986. *Necessary Losses*. New York: Ballantine Books.

SUGGESTED READING LIST

Anderson, Ray S. 1995. *Unspoken Wisdom – Truths My Father Taught Me.* Minneapolis: Augsburg.

Blauner, Bob. 1997. *Our Mothers' Spirits – On the Death of Mothers and the Grief of Men.* New York: Regan Books.

Bly, Robert. 1990. *Iron John.* Reading, MA: Addison.

Buscaglia, Leo. 1989. *Papa, My Father – A Celebration of Dads.* Thorofare, NJ: SLACK, Inc.

Campbell, Joseph. 1976. *The Portable Jung.* New York: Penguin Books.

Chethik, Neil. 2000. "Reaching Bereaved Men Requires Innovation," *The Forum*, September/October.

Chethik, Neil. 2001. *FatherLoss – How Sons of All Ages Come to Terms with the Deaths of their Dads.* New York: Hyperion.

Culbertson, Philip L. 1994. *Counseling Men.* Minneapolis: Fortress Press.

Doka, Kenneth. 1989. *Disenfranchised Grief: Recognizing Hidden Sorrow.* Lexington, MA: Lexington Press.

Doka, Kenneth, and Terry Martin. 2000. *Men Don't Cry...Women Do: Transcending Gender Stereotypes of Grief.* Bristol, PA: Taylor & Francis.

Gilligan, Carol, 1982. *In a Different Voice – Psychological Theory and Women's Development.* Cambridge: Harvard University Press.

Goebel, Julie. 1994. "Grief Experience Inventory," *GEI Review*, 4 (2). New Albany, IN.

Golden, Thomas R. 2000. *Swallowed by a Snake – The Gift of the Masculine Side of Healing*. Gaithersburg, MD: Golden Healing Publishing L.L.C.

Gray, John. 1992. *Men Are From Mars, Women Are From Venus*. New York: HarperCollins Publishers.

Gurian, Michael. 1993. *The Prince and The King – Healing the Father-Son Wound*. New York: Jeremy P. Tarcher/Perigee Books.

Heim, P., and S. Golant. 1992. *Hardball for Women: Winning at the Game of Business*. Los Angeles: Lowell House.

Hicks, Robert. 1991. *Uneasy Manhood*. Nashville: Oliver-Nelson Books.

Keen, Sam. 1992. *Fire in the Belly – On Being a Man*. New York: Bantam Books.

Keen, Sam. 1997. *To Love and Be Loved*. New York: Bantam Books.

Miller, James, and Thomas Golden. 1998. *A Man You Know Is Grieving/When a Man Faces Grief*. Fort Wayne: Willowgreen Publishing.

Moore, John H. 1989. *But What About Men – After Women's Lib*. Bath, Great Britain: Ashgrove Press Limited.

Moss, Miriam S., Sidney Z. Moss, and R. L. Rubinstein. 1996-97. "Middle-Aged Son's Reactions to Father's Death," *Omega* 34 (4): 259-277.

Nadeau, Janice Winchester. 1997. *Families Making Sense of Death.* Thousand Oaks, CA: Sage Publishers.

Pierce, Carol, and Bill Page. 1990. *A Male/Female Continuum: Paths to Colleagueship.* Laconia, NH: New Dynamics Publications.

Rando, Therese. 1986. *Parental Loss of a Child.* Champaign, IL: Research Press Company.

Rogness, Andrew. 1994. *Crossing Boundary Waters.* Minneapolis: Augsburg.

Rosenblatt, P. C., R. P. Walsh, and D. A. Jackson. 1976. *Grief and Mourning in Cross-Cultural Perspective.* H.R.A.F. Press.

Scull, Charles. 1992. *Fathers, Sons & Daughters – Exploring Fatherhood, Renewing the Bond.* New York: Jeremy P. Tarcher/Perigee Books.

Shapiro, Rami M. 1997. *Minyan – Ten Principles for Living a Life of Integrity.* New York: Bell Tower.

Somé, Malidoma Patrice. 1993. *Ritual: Power, Healing and Community.* Portland: Swan Raven and Company.

Staudacher, Carol. 1989. *Beyond Grief: A Guide for Recovering from the Death of a Loved One.* Oakland: New Harbinger Publications, Inc.

Staudacher, Carol. 1991. *Men and Grief.* Oakland: New Harbinger Publications, Inc.

Tannen, Deborah. 1990. *You Just Don't Understand – Women and Men in Conversation.* New York: Bantam Books.

Viorst, Judith. 1986. *Necessary Losses*. New York: Ballantine Books.